MW00389050

Psychiatric Pharmacogenomics

This material is not intended to be, and should not be considered, a substitute for medical or other professional advice. Treatment for the conditions described in this material is highly dependent on the individual circumstances. While this material is designed to offer accurate information with respect to the subject matter covered and to be current as of the time it was written, research and knowledge about medical and health issues is constantly evolving, and dose schedules for medications are being revised continually, with new side effects recognized and accounted for regularly. Readers must therefore always check the product information and clinical procedures with the most up-to-date published product information and data sheets provided by the manufacturers and the most recent codes of conduct and safety regulation. Oxford University Press and the author make no representations or warranties to readers, express or implied, as to the accuracy or completeness of this material, including without limitation that they make no representations or warranties as to the accuracy or efficacy of the drug dosages mentioned in the material. The author and the publishers do not accept, and expressly disclaim, any responsibility for any liability, loss, or risk that may be claimed or incurred as a consequence of the use and/or application of any of the contents of this material.

PSYCHIATRIC PHARMACOGENOMICS

David A. Mrazek, M.D., F.R.C.Psych.

Chair of Psychiatry and Psychology, Mayo Clinic
Professor of Psychiatry and Pediatrics
Mayo Clinic College of Medicine
Rochester, Minnesota

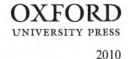

OXFORD
UNIVERSITY PRESS

2010

OXFORD
UNIVERSITY PRESS

Oxford University Press, Inc., publishes works that further
Oxford University's objective of excellence
in research, scholarship, and education.

Oxford   New York
Auckland   Cape Town   Dar es Salaam   Hong Kong   Karachi
Kuala Lumpur   Madrid   Melbourne   Mexico City   Nairobi
New Delhi   Shanghai   Taipei   Toronto

With offices in
Argentina   Austria   Brazil   Chile   Czech Republic   France   Greece
Guatemala   Hungary   Italy   Japan   Poland   Portugal   Singapore
South Korea   Switzerland   Thailand   Turkey   Ukraine   Vietnam

Copyright © 2010 by David A. Mrazek

Published by Oxford University Press, Inc.
198 Madison Avenue, New York, New York 10016

www.oup.com

Oxford is a registered trademark of Oxford University Press

All rights reserved. No part of this publication may be reproduced,
stored in a retrieval system, or transmitted, in any form or by any means,
electronic, mechanical, photocopying, recording, or otherwise,
without the prior permission of Oxford University Press.

Library of Congress Cataloging-in-Publication Data

Mrazek, David.
Psychiatric pharmacogenomics / by David A. Mrazek.
p.   ;   cm.
Includes bibliographical references and index.
ISBN 978-0-19-536729-4
1. Psychotropic drugs.   2. Pharmacogenomics.   I. Title.
[DNLM: 1. Biotransformation—genetics.   2. Psychotropic Drugs—adverse effects.
3. Mental Disorders—drug therapy.   4. Psychotropic Drugs—pharmacokinetics.
QV 38 M939p 2010]
RM315.M73 2010
615'.788—dc22
2009027407

ACKNOWLEDGMENTS

The creation of this book involved many people, and I am deeply grateful for the help that I have received over the three years that it took to conceptualize, compile, and craft this complicated collection of molecular variations, contradictory research findings, and intriguing clinical implications.

I had been planning to write this book for the past decade. As time passed, my motivation to make the book a reality intensified as I became increasingly aware of the importance of pharmacogenomics for the treatment of psychiatric patients.

I could not have written the book without many consultations with my colleagues to whom I owe much. I want to emphasize that many of the most valuable insights in the book were the result of these consultations. In contrast, the inevitable limitations of the book are the consequence of my own limitations in grasping the complexities of molecular human variation.

I am indebted to Marion Osmun of Oxford University Press for believing that the book would be important and persuading me that this was true. However, it took more than a year for a formal proposal to emerge and a contract to materialize. I was saddened when Marion decided to leave Oxford University Press, but relieved that she remained involved with the project. Subsequently, Shelley Reinhardt moved the project forward and then a year ago Craig Panner became involved in the production of the book and brought the project to its final conclusion.

Many friends, colleagues, and mentees read parts or all of the manuscript. I would like to extend thanks to Naleen Andrade, John L. Black, Janice Forster, Jim Kennedy, Barbara Koenig, Victor Reus, James Rundell, John Sadler, David Skuse, Rick Smith, Chris Wall, and Richard Weinshilboum for their help. A special thanks is due to Eric Wieben, a gifted scientist and teacher who carefully reviewed the entire manuscript to help me clarify the representations of components of the genes that are described in the book.

While I received ongoing support from all of the members of the Gene Team at the Mayo Clinic, special thanks must be extended to Barbara Hall who worked tirelessly to help me get the facts "right." Her attention to detail has been critical for ensuring the accuracy of the technical sections, gene maps, and references.

Finally, I would like to extend a special expression of thanks to my family. My four children, Nicola, Matthew, Michael and Alissa, each in their own way encouraged me to complete this project. However, it was my wife, Pat, who helped me find the hours to bring this project to completion and served as an ever-available and faithful sounding board to help me to think through the implications of pharmacogenomic translational research for clinical practice.

CONTENTS

VI. THE DOPAMINE RECEPTOR GENES

VII. CLINICAL CONSIDERATIONS

Fourteen Pharmacogenomically Relevant Genes

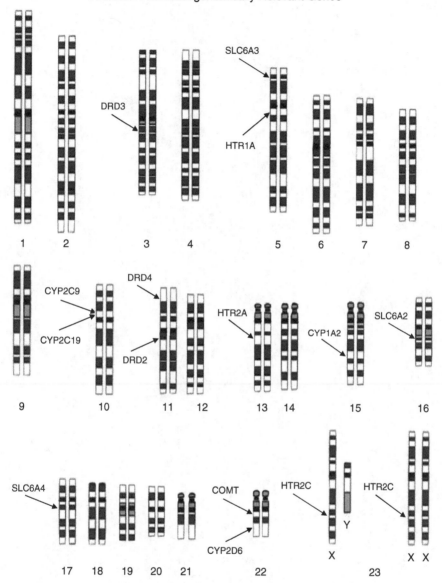

I
Basic Foundations

INTRODUCTION

Psychiatric pharmacogenomics is the study of how gene variations influence the responses of a patient to treatment with psychotropic medications. There are two primary goals of psychiatric pharmacogenomics in clinical practice. The first objective is to use information about structural gene variants to minimize the potential adverse effects of psychotropic medications. The second objective is to be able to use genetic testing to identify specific psychotropic medications that will have a high probability of being effective for an individual patient. The achievement of these goals has made it possible to begin to practice individualized molecular medicine. While the benefits of individualized medicine will positively influence all medical specialties, "there is no specialty where the need seems more compelling than for psychiatry" (Pickar, 2003).

The scientific foundation of the field of psychiatric pharmacogenomics has evolved over the past 30 years. This progress has been the consequence of a complex series of research developments that have included detailed studies of both the pharmacokinetics and the pharmacodynamics of psychotropic medications. Pharmacokinetics is the study of how drugs are metabolized, and provides information about the availability of a medication at the target site of the drug. Pharmacodynamics is the study of drug action at the target site of the drug.

The clinical implementation of psychiatric pharmacogenomic testing did not begin until 2003. The adoption of clinical psychiatric pharmacogenomic genotyping was accelerated in 2004 by the introduction of a U.S. Food and Drug Administration (FDA-) approved methodology for ascertaining the genotypes of two well-studied cytochrome P450 enzyme genes. Within the context of an increasingly broad concern about the safety of psychotropic medications, the field of clinical psychiatric pharmacogenomics has begun to expand. Furthermore, it is widely anticipated that with the additional testing of each new informative gene variant, the clinical utility of pharmacogenomic genotyping will inevitably increase (Mrazek, 2006).

This book is written for clinicians who prescribe psychotropic medications to treat targeted psychiatric symptoms. Given that antidepressants are the most commonly prescribed medications in the United States (Paulose-Ram et al., 2007), improving the outcome of using these medications is of interest to virtually all practicing psychiatrists, as well as an increasingly large number of primary care practitioners and clinical nurse specialists. Moreover, developing new methodologies to enhance the safety of prescribing psychotropic medications has become an increasingly high priority due to a greater appreciation of the serious adverse events that have been associated with the use of these medications. This increase in concern has been clearly highlighted by a series of FDA black-box warnings over the past several years.

STRATEGIES FOR READING THIS BOOK

A central objective of this book is to describe the clinical indications for the genetic tests that are currently available to clinicians and to review how the results of these tests can be used to improve the treatment that clinicians provide their patients. Consequently, the book has been designed in a manner that makes it possible to be read in three quite different ways.

The first way to read this book is to focus primarily on the clinical sections in each of the chapters that describe a single gene (i.e., Chapters 4–17). Each of these 14 chapters discusses the clinical implications of genotyping that specific gene, and defines the specific gene variations that have been associated with key clinical phenotypes. While quite detailed technical information about these gene variations is included in a special section in each chapter, those clinicians who are primarily interested in using the results of clinical pharmacogenomic testing to treat their patients can focus on the explanation of the test results and on the clinical vignettes that illustrate common treatment considerations. These vignettes are cumulative: that is, once a variant has been described in a chapter, consequences of testing that gene may be included in subsequent chapters and vignettes. Therefore, vignettes in later chapters include more pharmacogenomic genetic variants than do the vignettes in earlier chapters.

A second way to read this book is to focus on the in-depth discussions of the overall structure and the informative genetic variations of the 14 genes described in Chapters 4 through 17. For the clinician who wants to develop a deeper understanding of the specific gene variations and their clinical significance for the designation of phenotypes, each of these chapters describes the structure of a given gene and discusses how variability within the structure of that gene leads to changes in the amount of gene product that is available or in the function of the protein that is produced by the gene. Readers with an academic interest in psychiatric pharmacogenomics will find that these reviews provide them with a new opportunity to better understand the mechanisms by which genotyping defines the function of each of these genes. Quite technical information is included in these sections. Much of this technical information has not been previously published in either psychiatric journals or psychiatric textbooks. A detailed "map" of the clinically relevant variants for each of these genes is also included in these sections, and the structural changes that define these variants are explicitly described. Importantly, as appropriate in many of these chapters, the unique reference sequence number (i.e., rs number) of each variant is documented. The rs number is a unique identifier assigned by the National Center for Biotechnology Information (NCBI) and refers to a single nucleotide polymorphism (SNP). The rs number is sometimes called the "rsSNP ID" or "refSNP."

In addition to providing the unique rs number, which has become the current standard methodology for labeling SNPs, many of these chapters mention the previous idiosyncratic names or aliases that have been given to these variants. An "alias" can consist of the nucleotide change and the nucleotide location that has been used historically to define a polymorphism. Alternatively, an alias can consist of the amino acid change and the position of that change in the sequence of the amino acids that make up the peptide that is produced by the gene. Finally, the idiosyncratic names for the oldest variants that were first described in the pioneering studies of pharmacogenomics are also included. Taking the time to read these more in-depth technical discussions of how structural variations influence gene function will enable the reader to better understand the quite turgid technical reports in the scientific literature. It will also provide insights into the scientific rationale for clinical genotyping.

The third way to use this book is as a reference text. Even after mastering the basic rationale and indications for genetic testing, most practitioners will still find it helpful to have a handy reference available to look up the clinical implications of their patients' laboratory results. While a number of websites exist that contain relevant information for the clinical interpretation of specific genotypes, many of these online resources are not very user friendly. Consequently, busy clinicians may prefer to turn to an efficient and familiar reference to refresh their memories of the clinical implications of the most common gene variations. Specifically, they may find the succinct descriptions of the probable clinical implications of specific genotypes that are included in these chapters to be particularly useful at the time that they receive a new laboratory report. This will become increasingly important as patients begin to expect that their genotype results will be used to guide the treatment decisions of their physicians. The book is thus designed to help clinicians effectively explain the implications of identified genetic variants to their patients as one component of their clinical evaluations. Each chapter is organized in a consistent manner in order to facilitate the use of the book as an efficient reference.

CHAPTER OVERVIEWS

The first chapter in this book reviews the basic language of molecular genetics, with the goal of orienting the reader to key concepts associated with gene structure and function. Chapter 2 discusses how the genes reviewed in the book are similar and different from each other. The variation in their size and complexity indicates the range of variability in these important genes that can influence thought, emotions, and behavior. Chapter 3 illustrates the clinical utility of pharmacogenomic testing in practice and reviews the testing of a single family. Although the members of this family have relatively common genotypes, pharmacogenomic testing sheds light on how to effectively select appropriate psychotropic medications to manage their respective psychiatric problems.

As noted previously, Chapters 4 through 17 are each devoted to a discussion of a single gene that is currently being genotyped to guide clinical practice. These chapters begin with a brief contextual discussion about a given gene—for example, about its original discovery or the primary utiliza-tion of its genotyping in clinical practice. The chromosomal location of the gene is then identified, and a figure is provided that shows the specific chromosome where the gene is found and the precise location of the gene on that chromosome. This is followed by a map of the gene, including those gene variations believed to have the most significant effect on the function of the gene. The next section in each of these "single-gene" chapters includes a "technical discussion" of the variability that occurs within each of the specific genes. This discussion focuses on those variations that are being identified by clinical laboratories, because these variants have been asso-ciated with specific drug responses. A standard description of the most clinically relevant alleles for the gene is provided, with attention to why these particular gene variations are clinically important. Where appropriate, a standard table is included that identifies the specific nucleotide variations that define each mutant allele. The next section in these 14 chapters reviews the implications of the geographic ancestry of patients. Geographic ancestral variations in allele frequencies are particularly important for those genes that have the highest degree of structural variability. This is well illustrated in the discussion of the cytochrome P450 2D6 gene (Chapter 4). The subsequent section in these chapters highlights the specific genotypes that are associated with atypical patterns of drug response. These different patterns of response are often referred to as *clinical phenotypes*. The clinical phenotypes of the drug-metabolizing enzyme genes are often referred to as the ultra-rapid, normal, intermediate, and poor metabolizer phenotypes (Chapters 4–7). A quite practical section in these chapters is the discussion of the clinical indications for genotyping a specific gene. This includes how gene variations affect the metabolism of specific medications or predict variability in the effects of these drugs. Each of these chapters thus focuses, as warranted, on how antidepressants, antipsychotics, and other psychotropic medications are affected by the variations in the gene being discussed. Other selected medications and substances that are influenced by variation in the gene are also discussed, to help clinicians develop a better understanding of possible drug–drug interactions that can be complicated by genetic variation.

Next, vignettes that illustrate the clinical use of pharmacogenomic testing are usually included in each chapter. These pharmacogenomic test reports get gradually more complex as the reader is introduced to the series of informative pharmacogenomic genotypes. Finally, key clinical considerations are summarized at the end of each of these 14 chapters.

Medical investigators and clinicians have been grappling with how to best quantify the clinical utility of pharmacogenomic testing in order to achieve a consensus regarding how best to use this testing to guide treatment. Chapter 18 reviews the clinical utilization of genotyping and puts forward a rationale for how testing can improve practice by systematically calculating the probabilities of how specific gene variations may be associated with better medication response.

Chapter 19 highlights some of the key ethical questions related to the use of clinical genotyping. The basic conclusion of the chapter is that, while using pharmacogenomic data raises many issues that affect the care of patients, these are essentially the same considerations that are raised by any clinically informative laboratory data. The chapter identifies four key principles that are generally helpful to consider in assessing the appropriateness of clinical genotyping in the practice of psychiatry.

The final chapter of the book looks into the future. One major issue will be how to develop bioinformatics strategies to help clinicians manage the enormous amount of new clinical data that is becoming available to them. Nonetheless, the future development of psychiatric pharmacogenomics promises to make it possible for clinicians, through extensive genotyping, to practice much more effectively because of their being able to apply more individualized strategies in the care of their patients. The goal of prescribing the right drug for the right patient at the right dose is clearly in sight.

REFERENCES

Mrazek, D. (2006). Psychiatric Pharmacogenomics. *Focus, IV*(3), 1–5.

Paulose-Ram, R., Safran, M. A., Jonas, B. S., Gu, Q., & Orwig, D. (2007). Trends in psychotropic medication use among U.S. adults. *Pharmacoepidemiology & Drug Safety, 16*(5), 560–570.

Pickar, D. (2003). Pharmacogenomics of psychiatric drug treatment. *Psychiatric Clinics of North America, 26*(2), 303–321.

1

THE LANGUAGE OF MOLECULAR GENETICS

The world of the molecular geneticist is composed of many different varieties of "gene maps." These gene maps represent an entirely different genre of cartography than most physicians have mastered. Amazingly, these maps are constructed by what seems to be endless sequences of the all-important four nucleotides that are the basic building blocks of gene structure: adenine, cytosine, guanine, and thymine.

Adding to this complexity is the language of molecular genetics itself, which includes hundreds of cryptic abbreviations and technical terms. For example, the abbreviation 5-HTTLPR is just one of several names that describe a single specific gene variation that is more accurately described as the "indel" promoter polymorphism of the serotonin transporter gene, SLC6A4. However, to conserve space in scientific reports, molecular geneticists have created a shorthand methodology for communicating about genes that is difficult for most physicians to comprehend. What has emerged are "dialects" of the language of molecular genetics that are inscrutable to many psychiatrists who have not had the opportunity to understand how gene variations may ultimately influence the responses of their patients to standard medication treatment.

It is also true that psychiatrists have their own language to describe the phenotypes of their patients and the treatments that they provide to them. For example, psychiatric clinicians still debate the importance of specific diagnostic criteria for a patient who presents with a provisional diagnosis of schizoaffective disorder with grandiose delusions. These patients are characterized by psychotic thinking and depressive symptoms. However, these same symptoms are components of the diagnostic criteria for bipolar disorder. Unfortunately, many molecular geneticists, as well as other medical colleagues, have little appreciation of the essence of these diagnostic debates. The dilemma of cross-discipline communication becomes even more problematic when psychiatrists begin to speculate on how environmental and interpersonal influences may increase the risk for akathisia in a patient who is treated with olanzapine versus perphenazine. Almost all comprehension is lost when shorthand terms are used, such as referring to the "CATIE study" (Clinical Antipsychotic Trials of Intervention Effectiveness) as the primary source of evidence that makes it possible to balance the benefits of these medications (e.g., the relief of primary symptoms) with their potential risk (e.g., development of metabolic syndrome) (Lieberman et al., 2005). The reality is that most molecular geneticists and even many primary care physicians who prescribe antipsychotic medications have never heard of the CATIE study.

A core goal of this book is to provide a "bridge" between these two worlds and to translate the language of molecular genetics for psychiatrists, so that they can access the world of pharmacogenomics. This chapter aims to give clinicians enough understanding of the basics of this language to enable them to appreciate the detailed descriptions of the structures of the genes reviewed in this volume. Simply stated, its objective is to briefly discuss the ways in which molecular geneticists describe genes.

Of course, this short chapter will not provide the reader a deep understanding of how genes work. The goal of the chapter is much more modest. Ultimately, the point of learning this language is to gain a better understanding of how variations in gene structure are linked to gene function and why some patients respond differently to psychotropic medications than do others.

DESCRIBING THE STRUCTURE OF A GENE

To understand the structural changes in genes described in this book, it is necessary to master some elementary vocabulary. Genes are located on *chromosomes*. There are 23 pairs of chromosomes. Twenty-two of these pairs are described as *autosomes*. The final pair consists of two sex chromosomes. Women have two copies of the X chromosome. Men have one copy of the X chromosome and one copy of the Y chromosome.

Every chromosome has a short arm and long arm separated by a *centromere*, which is a central constriction within the body of the chromosome. The longer arm of the chromosome is called the *q arm*. The shorter arm is referred to as the *p arm*. The chromosomal *locus* of a gene is the particular position of a gene on the chromosome. An example of how the position of a gene is designated is 1p13.2. The first number refers to the number of the

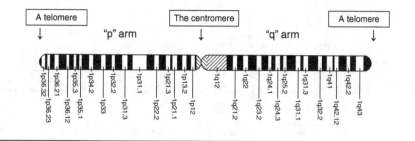

FIGURE 1.1. An illustration of chromosome 1 and its component parts.

chromosome. The p refers to the short arm. The second number refers to the region or "cytogenetic band" of the chromosome where the gene is located. The *telomeres* are located at the two ends of each chromosome. Figure 1.1 is an illustration of chromosome 1, showing its most basic component parts.

A gene is essentially a long sequence of four different nucleotides. The variation in the sequence of these four nucleotides defines approximately 20,500 genes that code for more than 100,000 proteins. Again, these four nucleotides are adenine, cytosine, guanine, and thymine. They are universally referred to as A, C, G, and T. Adenine and guanine are purines. Cytosine and thymine are pyrimidines (Clamp et al., 2007).

The length of a gene can vary dramatically. The smallest genes are composed of less than 1,000 nucleotides. Large genes can extend well beyond a million nucleotides. However, regardless of the length of the gene, its coding sequences are made up of one or more series of *triplets* composed of three nucleotides. Each triplet defines a single *codon*. The codons are included within those portions of the gene that are designated as *exons*. An exon is a segment that is represented in the final mRNA product of a gene. In more evolved genes, there may be many exons, whereas in the most primitive genes only one exon exists. The nucleotides between any two exons are referred to as an *intron*. The functions of the nucleotides that make up the intron are still not well understood, although it is increasingly clear that some of these nucleotide sequences play a role in gene regulation and gene expression.

A gene map is traditionally organized with the 5' FR (i.e., five-prime flanking region) located to the left of the start codon. The nucleotides in this region are not transcribed and do not code for amino acids. The 3' FR (i.e., three-prime flanking region) is traditionally located on the right of the gene map. The nucleotides in this region also are not transcribed and do not code for amino acids. Protein coding genes also have regions called "untranslated regions" at both ends. These are transcribed, but these "leader" and "trailer" sequences do not code for amino acids. Figure 1.2 illustrates a gene map that designates both the 5' FR and the 3' FR.

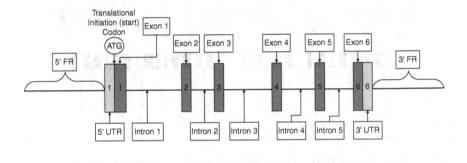

FIGURE 1.2. Illustration of a generic gene map.

The *start codon* is designated by three nucleotides that are conventionally labeled as nucleotide 1, nucleotide 2, and nucleotide 3. The first exon usually begins before the start codon or initiation codon. In DNA, this start codon includes the nucleotides adenine, thymine, and guanine, and is abbreviated ATG. The nucleotide locations that are represented to the left of the start codon are assigned negative numbers and are described as being "upstream" of the start codon. The nucleotides that extend to the right of the start codon are described as being "downstream," toward the 3' region of the gene. Genes have a *promoter region* that is found upstream of the start codon. A promoter is a region of DNA that facilitates the transcription of a particular gene. Basic promoters are typically located in the 5' flanking region of the genes that they regulate. By convention, nucleotides that make up the promoter region are given negative numbers.

DESCRIBING GENE VARIATION

Gene variations are among the most essential biological differences that define individual variability. The simplest gene variation is the substitution of one nucleotide for another. This is referred to as a *single nucleotide polymorphism* (SNP). The choice of the term *polymorphism* is unfortunate, because it literally means "many shapes" rather than "single substitution." However, "single nucleotide polymorphism" is now a core term in the language of molecular genetics. The technical definition of a SNP is a single nucleotide substitution that occurs in a population at a frequency of at least 1%. If a single nucleotide substitution occurs less frequently than in 1% of the population, it is technically referred to as a *mutation*. Again, this is an unfortunate term to have been chosen to describe these less-common variants because there are many other uses of the term "mutation" that have little to do with SNPs.

A SNP can occur within a codon. If the SNP results in the codon coding for a different amino acid, it is described as a *nonsynonymous SNP*. If the codon still codes for the same amino acid despite the nucleotide substitution, it is described as a *synonymous SNP*. The intronic regions of the gene are, by definition, regions not involved in coding. In Chapters 8 through 17, SNPs will be identified by using their unique reference sequence number, which is also called the *rs number*. However, many famous SNPs, such as the Val variant and Met variant of the catechol-O-methyltransferase gene (i.e., COMT) are known primarily by their idiosyncratic popular name. These and other aliases will be defined in the more technical section of each chapter that describes a specific gene.

Another common gene variation is the *insertion* of one or more nucleotides into the coding region of the gene. Insertions that consist of three nucleotides or a multiple of three nucleotides usually have less effect on the gene product because the consequence of these insertions is limited to the addition of either one or a small number of amino acids. If the insertion is less than three nucleotides or not a multiple of three nucleotides, the consequence is a *frame shift mutation*, which almost universally results in a gene product that is not functional because most of the downstream amino acids are altered.

The same principles must be considered when nucleotides are *deleted* from a codon. A structural change in the sequence results when one or more nucleotides are deleted. If the deletion consists of three nucleotides or a multiple of three nucleotides, again, no frame shift impact occurs on the gene product. In recent years, the abbreviation "indel" has been used generically to refer to either an insertion or a deletion.

CONCLUSION

Reading more about molecular genetics is strongly advised. A good place to start is to read *Genome* (2000) by Matt Ridley. A more up-to-date review of psychiatric genetics can be found in a text by Smoller et al. (2008). Readers should also refer to the extensive glossary at the end of this book, which is designed to help decode more technical descriptions of genes and their function.

REFERENCES

Clamp, M., Fry, B., Kamal, M., Xie, X., Cuff, J., Lin, M. F., et al. (2007). Distinguishing protein-coding and noncoding genes in the human genome. *Proceedings of the National Academy of Sciences of the United States of America, 104*(49), 19428–19433.

Lieberman, J. A., Stroup, T. S., McEvoy, J. P., Swartz, M. S., Rosenheck, R. A., Perkins, D. O., et al., CATIE Investigators. (2005). Effectiveness of antipsychotic drugs in patients with chronic schizophrenia. *New England Journal of Medicine, 353*(12), 1209–1223.

Ridley, M. (2000). *Genome: the autobiography of a species in 23 chapters.* New York: HarperCollins.

Smoller, J. W., Shiedley, B. Rosen, T., & Ming T. (2008). *Psychiatric Genetics: applications in clinical practice.* Arlington: American Psychiatric Publishing, Inc.

2

The Fourteen Genes

In many ways, this book is the story of the variations in 14 different genes that influence how individual patients respond to specific psychotropic medications. The decision to include these particular genes was based on the practical consideration that, at least for the moment, these are the genes that clinical laboratories most commonly genotype to improve patient care. Because an increasingly large number of patients are being genotyped to define variations in these genes, it has become important for clinicians to understand what the implications of these variations are for the therapeutic responses of their patients. However, in the very near future, it will be imperative for clinicians to learn about variations in many more genes.

Introduction to the Fourteen Genes

The official names and abbreviations for these 14 genes are listed in Table 2.1 in the order that they appear in this book. The first two genes, cytochrome P450 2D6 gene (CYP2D6) and cytochrome P450 2C19 gene (CYP2C19) have been routinely tested in psychiatric practice since 2003. Consequently, many patients have already been tested for these two genes. Those patients who have either impaired or accelerated metabolism for 2D6 or 2C19 substrate medications have learned to be careful when using these drugs. An extensive explanation of the CYP2D6 gene variations and a clinical vignette is included in Chapter 4. Discussion of the CYP2C19 gene is given in Chapter 5.

The cytochrome P450 2C9 gene (CYP2C9) and the cytochrome P450 1A2 gene (CYP1A2) are described in Chapters 6 and 7, respectively. The

TABLE 2.1. Full names and abbreviations of the 14 genes

Complete Name	Abbreviation
Cytochrome P450 2D6 gene	CYP2D6
Cytochrome P450 2C19 gene	CYP2C19
Cytochrome P450 2C9 gene	CYP2C9
Cytochrome P450 1A2 gene	CYP1A2
Catecholamine-O-methyltransferase gene	COMT
Norepinephrine transporter gene	SLC6A2
Dopamine transporter gene	SLC6A3
Serotonin transporter gene	SLC6A4
Serotonin 1A receptor gene	HTR1A
Serotonin 2A receptor gene	HTR2A
Serotonin 2C receptor gene	HTR2C
D2 dopamine receptor gene	DRD2
D3 dopamine receptor gene	DRD3
D4 dopamine receptor gene	DRD4

CYP2C9 chapter focuses specifically on the value of testing this gene in patients who have an intermediate or poor 2D6 phenotype and describes the importance of testing the CYP2C9 gene in patients who require anti-coagulation treatment with warfarin. The CYP1A2 chapter focuses on the importance of the induction of the *1F variant by the use of tobacco and reviews the implication of this variant for the metabolism of clozapine, olanzapine, and fluvoxamine, as well as other psychotropic medications for which CYP1A2 plays a role in metabolism.

The catecholamine-O-methyltransferase gene (COMT) has been extensively studied. However, the focus of the review of COMT in Chapter 8 is primarily on the pharmacogenomic implications of COMT variability.

Three neurotransmitter transporter genes are reviewed in Chapters 9 through 11. An understanding of the functional variations in these genes is still evolving. Furthermore, the implications of the variations in the transporter genes have not been systematically incorporated into clinical practice guidelines. However, the importance of the genetic variations in these genes is becoming better understood, and the clinical implications of these variations are reviewed and summarized. Moreover, the serotonin transporter gene (SLC6A4) has been extensively studied, and the clinical implications for antidepressant treatments in patients having alleles that produce more serotonin transporter protein are reviewed. Variations in the dopamine transporter gene (SLC6A3) and the norepinephrine transporter gene (SLC6A2) are also discussed within the context of making pharmacogenomically informed clinical decisions.

Chapters 12 through 17 describe six neurotransmitter receptor genes, focusing primarily on the pharmacogenomic implications of gene variations rather than on the implications of these variations for disease expression. However, some associations between gene variations and psychopathology are reviewed.

LOCATION AND SIZE OF THE FOURTEEN GENES

Table 2.2 reveals the specific chromosomal location of each of the 14 pharmacogenomically informative genes. The distribution of these genes across the chromosomes is not random. For example, both CYP2D6 and COMT are located on the smallest autosome, chromosome 22. Somewhat surprisingly, none of these 14 genes is located on either chromosome 1 or chromosome 2, which are the two largest chromosomes. However, the implications of the chromosomal location of these genes are still not well understood.

The 14 genes vary dramatically in size. Table 2.3 lists the genes by their size, as measured by the number of nucleotides within each gene. The largest is the serotonin 2C receptor gene (HTR2C), which has 326,074 nucleotides. In contrast, the serotonin 1A receptor gene (HTR1A) has only 1,269 nucleotides.

These 14 genes also vary quite dramatically in their complexity, as illustrated in Table 2.4. HTR1A has only one exon whereas SLC6A4 and SLC6A3 each have 15 exons.

Although these genes vary greatly in size and complexity, their protein gene products are actually quite similar in size, as illustrated in Table 2.5. The gene that produces the largest protein product is SLC6A4, which produces a protein containing 630 amino acids. In contrast, the COMT protein product is less than half the size of the SLC6A4 protein product and is composed of only 271 amino acids.

TABLE 2.2. The 14 genes and their chromosomal location

Gene	Chromosomal Location
CYP2D6	22q13.1
CYP2C19	10q24.1-q24.3
CYP2C9	10q24
CYP1A2	15q24
COMT	22q11.21
SLC6A2	16q12.2
SLC6A3	5p15.3
SLC6A4	17q11.1-q12
HTR1A	5q11.2-q13
HTR2A	13q14-q21
HTR2C	Xq24
DRD2	11q23
DRD3	3q13.3
DRD4	11p15.5

TABLE 2.3. The size of the 14 genes as measured by the number of nucleotides within each gene

Gene	# of Nucleotides
HTR1A	1269
DRD4	3399
CYP2D6	4383
CYP1A2	7758
COMT	27222
SLC6A4	37800
SLC6A2	47145
DRD3	50343
CYP2C9	50708
SLC6A3	52637
HTR2A	62663
DRD2	65565
CYP2C19	90209
HTR2C	326074

TABLE 2.4. The complexity of the 14 genes as measured by the number of exons

Gene	# of Exons
HTR1A	1
HTR2A	3
DRD4	4
COMT	6
HTR2C	6
CYP1A2	7
DRD2	8
DRD3	8
CYP2D6	9
CYP2C9	9
CYP2C19	9
SLC6A2	14
SLC6A4	15
SLC6A3	15

TABLE 2.5. The size of the protein gene products that are coded for by these 14 genes

Gene	# of Amino Acids
COMT	271
DRD3	367
DRD4	419
HTR1A	422
DRD2	443
HTR2C	458
HTR2A	471
CYP2C9	490
CYP2C19	490
CYP2D6	497
CYP1A2	516
SLC6A2	617
SLC6A3	620
SLC6A4	630

CONCLUSION

These 14 pharmacogenomically relevant genes all play important roles in either the pharmacokinetic availability of psychotropic drugs or their pharmacodynamic effects. Variations in the structures of the drug-metabolizing genes are potentially important predictors of pharmacokinetic differences. Variations in the transporter and receptor genes can lead to the development of symptoms that may benefit from psychotropic medications or may actually modulate the pharmacodynamic responses of patients who are receiving psychotropic medication.

For reasons that are not well understood, these genes are not evenly distributed across the 23 chromosomes. Furthermore, while the 14 genes overviewed here vary enormously in size, the size of the proteins that they code for are actually quite similar. Finally, the complexities of these genes vary dramatically from simple to highly evolved. Future research efforts will hopefully shed greater light on the significance of these differences.

3

THE PROBLEM AND THE SOLUTION

A basic problem for psychiatrists is how to more effectively select psychotropic drugs that can relieve their patients' symptoms without causing uncomfortable and potentially dangerous adverse effects. Pharmacogenomic testing provides a new tool to help solve this problem, as it gives clinicians highly reliable, individualized genomic information about their patients that makes it possible for them to select medications with a higher probability of achieving a successful outcome and a lower risk of their patients developing side effects.

The adverse effects of psychotropic drugs are a major concern. Common side effects of the antidepressants include headache, nausea, diarrhea, and problems with sexual function. All of these side effects have a negative impact on adherence. Furthermore, the activation of mania or the potentiation of suicidal ideation have been associated with the use of antidepressants and can have lethal consequences. Serious side effects of antipsychotic medications include obesity, metabolic syndrome, diabetes, and extrapyramidal symptoms. Chronic exposure to both typical and atypical antipsychotic medications can also result in the development of tardive dyskinesia and permanent disability. Pharmacogenomic testing provides practical information that can be used to minimize the development of these adverse effects.

The benefits of pharmacogenomic testing are illustrated by the following analysis of the clinical care provided to the O'Brien family. A comprehensive discussion of the four genes that were tested during the course of this illustration can be found in Chapters 4–7. However, the goal of this illustration is to highlight the benefit of pharmacogenomic testing, rather than to describe variability in the structure and function of these four drug-metabolizing enzyme genes.

The O'Brien Family

Mr. William O'Brien

Mr. William O'Brien is a 43-year-old man of European ancestry who lives in Raleigh, North Carolina. He graduated from Duke University with a degree in chemistry. He married his wife shortly after his graduation, then began working for Dow Chemical, where he has remained employed for the past 20 years. At the age of 27, he developed a serious depression at the time of the death of his mother, who was killed instantly in a car accident. He was successfully treated with 20 mg of paroxetine, which was prescribed by his internist because he refused to consult a psychiatrist. After 2 years, his paroxetine treatment was discontinued. He subsequently remained free of depressive symptoms.

Mrs. Wendy O'Brien

Mrs. Wendy O'Brien is a 42-year-old woman of European ancestry who met her husband while she was a student at the University of North Carolina. She is a devout Christian who has committed herself to caring for their two sons, who are fraternal twins and were born 2 years after the O'Brien's married. Although Mrs. O'Brien did have symptoms of postpartum depression after the birth of the twins, her symptoms resolved spontaneously within 2 weeks of their delivery. She attributed her recovery to her own prayers and the prayers of her close friends.

When her sons left home during their junior year of high school to participate in a foreign exchange program in Spain, Mrs. O'Brien decided to look for a job to help pay for her sons' future college expenses. In October, she developed increasing difficulty with sleeping and a diminished appetite. She subsequently found it difficult to complete job applications and in November she stopped attending church services. She did feel somewhat better over the December holidays when her sons came home from Spain to celebrate Christmas. However, in January, she became even more acutely depressed and did not want to leave her house.

William ultimately took his wife to see their internist, who insisted that she be evaluated by a psychiatrist, Dr. Wanda Engel. Dr. Engel made the diagnosis of a major depressive disorder and prescribed 50 mg of fluvoxamine to be taken in the evening. Mrs. O'Brien reported limited improvement in her symptoms over the next 4 weeks, and Dr. Engel subsequently increased her dose of fluvoxamine to 100 mg taken in the evening. This increase in dose resulted in some nausea and a sense of restlessness, but Mrs. O'Brien continued to take her medication. After 8 weeks of treatment, her depressive symptoms were resolved. She subsequently felt a renewed sense of optimism, actively engaged in seeking employment, and was hired by the Raleigh Public Library as an assistant librarian in April.

George O'Brien

George O'Brien was always described by his mother as being the "good twin." He did well in school and was an accomplished competitive swimmer on the high school swim team. George experienced no early developmental difficulties and was a very healthy child. In the fall of his senior year, he applied to the early admission program at Stanford University. Given his good academic performance and his exceptional swimming record, he was not surprised that he was accepted at Stanford.

Shortly after his acceptance to Stanford, George started to become depressed and refused to go to school. Dr. Engel, who had treated his mother, evaluated George and felt that he could benefit from antidepressant medication. The plan that Dr. Engel developed was to treat George with either paroxetine or fluvoxamine, given that these medications had helped George's parents to recover from their earlier depressive illnesses. Her ultimate decision was to prescribe paroxetine for George, as Mr. O'Brien had done well when he was treated with this medication as a young man. Unfortunately, George had no therapeutic response to 20 mg of paroxetine. He became increasingly depressed and began to talk about quitting the swimming team. While his parents insisted that he continue to swim on the team, they became increasingly worried when his swimming performance began to deteriorate. After 4 weeks, his dose of paroxetine was increased to 40 mg. Over the next month, he reported no improvement in his symptoms, and he was consistently waking at 4:00 in the morning. Additionally, his teachers became concerned that he was no longer completing his homework.

Dr. Engel decided to discontinue George's paroxetine treatment and to initiate a course of fluvoxamine, given that Mrs. O'Brien had continued to do well taking fluvoxamine. George was initially prescribed 50 mg of fluvoxamine. After 4 weeks, George was enjoying some improvement in his depressive symptoms and started dating a classmate. However, he complained of persistent nausea, and fluvoxamine treatment was subsequently discontinued in April. By the beginning of May, George's depressive symptoms were returning. His parents were worried that if his depression again became severe, he might drop out of school. Dr. Engel suggested that venlafaxine would be a good alternative antidepressant, but George refused to take a third medication. Instead, he was willing to try transcranial magnetic stimulation. After 1 week of treatment, he felt considerably better. After his fourth week of treatment, his symptoms were largely resolved, and he was able to spend the summer training with the Stanford swimming team in anticipation of swimming competitively during his freshman year at the university.

Henry O'Brien

Henry O'Brien was often referred to by his mother as the "dark twin." He was a good student, but he never was as academically successful as his brother, George. The twins swam together on the community swim team in junior high school, but Henry was not fast enough to make the high school team. He did try out for football, but he broke his ankle during his freshman year and was unable to make the team in his sophomore year. He found it difficult to apply to any universities at the beginning of his senior year of high school, but he did finally complete an application to Whittier College in California, where he was accepted.

During his last semester of high school, Henry avoided being with George, who had become very withdrawn. Instead, he tried to be with his friends as much as possible. He began to attend parties on the weekends and would drink as many as a dozen beers in an evening. He also began to smoke heavily, defying his parents, who insisted that he should not smoke.

Henry did poorly at Whittier and dropped out after his first year. He returned home to live with his family and tried to find a job. In November, he developed suicidal ideation and began to confide in his mother that he no longer wanted to live. He also began drinking heavily every night and increased his smoking to two packs of cigarettes a day. His parents persuaded Henry to see Dr. Engel, who was still treating his mother and was familiar with the ongoing treatment of his brother. Once again, paroxetine was chosen to treat his depressive symptoms because Mr. O'Brien had responded well to treatment with this medication as a young man. Henry was initially given 20 mg of paroxetine. For the first week, he felt that his depressive symptoms were improved, but he developed a persistent headache. His dose was subsequently decreased to 10 mg of paroxetine, and he felt that his mood was somewhat better. However, after a second week of persistently severe headaches, he refused to continue taking paroxetine. Dr. Engel once again felt that fluvoxamine would be a good second choice, given that Henry's mother was still successfully being treated with a moderate dose of this medication. Dr. Engel initiated treatment with fluvoxamine at a dose of 50 mg. After 4 weeks, there was no improvement, and Henry's dose was increased to 100 mg, at which point he reported some improved symptoms despite a sense of persistent hopelessness. After another month, Henry concluded that the fluvoxamine was not sufficiently helpful to warrant his continuing to take the medication. He stopped taking fluvoxamine and announced to his parents that he had decided to leave home to live with a friend. Shortly after leaving home, his drinking became increasingly out of control and he ultimately had a car accident while intoxicated. Two passengers were injured in the accident, and he was sentenced to be admitted to an alcohol treatment facility or spend 6 months in a minimum-security correctional facility. Henry chose treatment and was successful in achieving abstinence.

Dr. Engel Seeks Consultation

Dr. Engel was puzzled about the fact that the twins had done so poorly while taking the same selective serotonin reuptake inhibitors (SSRIs) that had worked so well for their parents. She subsequently sought consultation with a senior colleague, who had been in practice for many years and was reputed to be a talented psychotherapist. After Dr. Engel carefully reviewed her management of these confusing cases, her colleague stressed that the boys had been very competitive with their father and that he believed it would be difficult for them to accept the same treatment that their father had received, given their unresolved feelings about his continuous economic success. He also pointed out that George had initially done well on the same medication as his mother and that an increase in the boy's libido while taking fluvox-amine may have occurred within the context of his feeling emotionally closer to his mother, as they were receiving the same medication. This closeness may have triggered forbidden impulses, which resulted in his needing to distance himself from his mother and her medicine. While Dr. Engel accepted that these speculations could conceivably have contributed to the negative outcome of her treatment, she could not conclude that they provided a fully credible explanation for the poor therapeutic response of the twins.

Dr. Engel subsequently sought a consultation with a second colleague, who was on the faculty at the medical school. Her second consultant advised Dr. Engel to order pharmacogenomic testing to determine whether genetic variability could have contributed to the poor treatment outcomes that she had described. Dr. Engel agreed, contacted the parents and the twins, and ultimately ordered a panel of four cytochrome P450 drug-metabolizing enzyme genes for each of the boys. The results provided a quite plausible explanation for their negative reactions.

PHARMACOGENOMIC TESTING AND ANALYSES

George (Table 3.1) was an ultra-rapid metabolizer of 2D6 substrate medications, based on having three active copies of the CYP2D6 gene. However, he was a poor metabolizer of 1A2 substrate medications, based on having no active copy of the CYP1A2 gene. He was a normal metabolizer of 2C9 and 2C19 substrate medications. George was unlikely to have developed an adequate serum level of paroxetine at 40 mg, and clearly was unwilling to continue taking paroxetine after 2 months of unsuccessful treatment. Given that he was

TABLE 3.1. George's pharmacogenomic report

Pharmacogenomic Report of George O'Brien		
Gene	Genotype of Patient	Clinical Implication
CYP2D6	*1Dup/*1	Ultra-rapid CYP2D6 metabolizer
CYP2C19	*1/*1	Normal CYP2C19 metabolizer
CYP2C9	*1/*1	Normal CYP2C9 metabolizer
CYP1A2	*6/*6	Poor CYP1A2 metabolizer

a poor metabolizer of 1A2 substrate medications, it was likely that when taking fluvoxamine he quickly developed a high serum level that successfully blocked serotonin reuptake. Yet, this high serum level was also responsible for his intolerable side effects. George clearly did well when treated with transcranial magnetic stimulation, but this is a relatively expensive treatment that may not have been necessary if he had been treated with an antidepressant that he would have been able to tolerate, such as escitalopram or sertraline.

Henry (Table 3.2) was a poor metabolizer of 2D6 substrate medications, based on having no active alleles of the CYP2D6 gene. He was also a potentially ultra-rapid metabolizer of 1A2 substrate medications, based on being homozygous for the *1F inducible allele of the CYP1A2 gene. Like his brother, Henry was a normal metabolizer of 2C9 and 2C19 substrate medications. Given that he was a poor metabolizer of CYP2D6 substrate medications, a dose of 20 mg of paroxetine would have resulted in a rapid and sustained high serum level, which he did not tolerate. In addition, given that he had a genotype associated with ultra-rapid metabolism of 1A2 substrate medications and that he was smoking heavily, which further induced the production of the 1A2 enzyme, it is highly improbable that he would be able to achieve a therapeutic serum level of fluvoxamine at standard doses. Like George, Henry would have been likely to tolerate an antidepressant medication that was metabolized by 2C19. If he had received effective treatment for

TABLE 3.2. Henry's pharmacogenomic report

Pharmacogenomic Report of Henry O'Brien		
Gene	Genotype of Patient	Clinical Implication
CYP2D6	*4/*4	Poor CYP2D6 metabolizer
CYP2C19	*1/*1	Normal CYP2C19 metabolizer
CYP2C9	*1/*1	Normal CYP2C9 metabolizer
CYP1A2	*1F/*1F	Ultra-rapid CYP1A2 metabolizer

TABLE 3.3. Mr. O'Brien's pharmacogenomic report

Pharmacogenomic Report of Mr. O'Brien		
Gene	Genotype of Patient	Clinical Implication
CYP2D6	*1/*4	Intermediate CYP2D6 metabolizer
CYP2C19	*1/*1	Normal CYP2C19 metabolizer
CYP2C9	*1/*1	Normal CYP2C9 metabolizer
CYP1A2	*6/*1F	Intermediate CYP1A2 metabolizer

TABLE 3.4. Mrs. O'Brien's pharmacogenomic report

Pharmacogenomic Report of Mrs. O'Brien		
Gene	Genotype of Patient	Clinical Implication
CYP2D6	*1Dup/*4	Normal CYP2D6 metabolizer
CYP2C19	*1/*1	Normal CYP2C19 metabolizer
CYP2C9	*1/*1	Normal CYP2C9 metabolizer
CYP1A2	*6/*1F	Intermediate CYP1A2 metabolizer

his mood disorder, Henry may have been less vulnerable to developing a pattern of abusing alcohol.

Given these informative results, Mr. and Mrs. O'Brien became interested in obtaining their respective genotypes for these drug-metabolizing genes.

Mr. O'Brien (Table 3.3) was an intermediate metabolizer of 2D6 and 1A2 substrate medications, as well as a normal metabolizer of 2C9 and 2C19 substrate medications. These phenotypes are very compatible with his good response to relatively modest doses of paroxetine, given that it is metabolized primarily by the 2D6 enzyme.

Mrs. O'Brien (Table 3.4) was an intermediate metabolizer of 1A2 substrate medications and a normal metabolizer of 2D6, 2C9, and 2C19 substrate medications. These phenotypes are quite compatible with her good response to a relatively modest dose of fluvoxamine, given that it is metabolized primarily by the 1A2 enzyme.

THE GENETIC EXPLANATION

Dr. Engel was initially perplexed that fraternal twin brothers could have responded so differently to similar treatment. While intellectually she understood that the boys were no more biologically similar than any two brothers

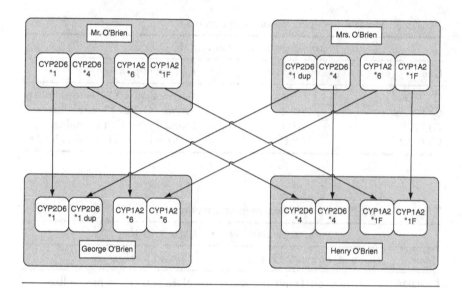

FIGURE 3.1. Illustration of the pattern of inheritance for CYP2D6 and CYP1A2 that resulted in the O'Brien twins' divergent genotypes.

were, ironically it seemed to her, on an emotional level, that they *should* be more similar. However, an analysis of the segregation of the CYP2D6 and CYP1A2 genes in the O'Brien family (Fig. 3.1) makes it quite clear that the brothers did not share any of their CYP2D6 or CYP1A2 genes. It also highlights the fact that it would have been impossible to accurately predict the genotypes of the boys based on the genotypes of the parents.

CONCLUSION

In retrospect, the treatment of the twins could have been both more effective and more affordable if they had been genotyped using a panel of cytochrome P450 genes prior to the onset of their treatment. Fortunately, because of genotyping, the family came to understand their capacities to metabolize medications, and the twins became more optimistic about their future prognosis and treatment.

II

THE DRUG-METABOLIZING ENZYME GENES

4

THE CYTOCHROME P450 2D6 GENE

Cytochrome P450 proteins have been classified and organized into families and subfamilies. These proteins all contain an iron or *heme* group; consequently, they are referred to as *hemoproteins*. The designation "cytochrome P450" refers to the fact that these proteins are colorful (i.e., *chromo*), because they contain pigment that absorbs light at approximately 450 nM wavelengths.

The cytochrome P450 2D6 gene (CYP2D6) was originally described as the debrisoquine 4-hydroxylase gene (Dayer et al., 1987; Kimura et al., 1989). This original name was chosen because the enzyme produced by this gene had been demonstrated to be necessary for the hydroxylation of the drug debrisoquine. Debrisoquine was an early antihypertensive medication that is no longer available for use in the United States because other antihypertensive medications have been developed that are more effective and have fewer side effects. Given that debrisoquine is no longer used, the original name for this enzyme, debrisoquine hydroxylase, has become an anachronism. However, the importance of this enzyme has become increasingly clear, as it is involved in the metabolism of more than 70 currently available medications. Once it was recognized that this enzyme was a member of the cytochrome P450 family of enzymes, debrisoquine hydroxylase was renamed using the P450 nomenclature. This enzyme is now routinely referred to as the cytochrome 2D6 enzyme or more simply as the 2D6 enzyme.

In addition to normal alleles that code for functional 2D6 enzyme, many inactive forms of CYP2D6 exist. These inactive forms of CYP2D6 are referred to as *inactive alleles* or *null alleles*. Some forms of the CYP2D6 gene also produce a form of the protein that has limited enzymatic activity. These partially active forms of CYP2D6 are usually called *deficient alleles*. Patients who only have inactive alleles do not produce any active 2D6 enzyme and consequently do not effectively metabolize 2D6 substrate medications. Conversely, patients with three or more active alleles are unlikely to benefit from treatment with 2D6 substrate medications, because they produce such an increased quantity of the 2D6 enzyme that they do not achieve adequate serum levels of the medication and do not benefit from taking these medications at traditional doses.

Location and Gene Variation

The CYP2D6 gene is located on chromosome 22, which is the smallest autosome. The specific location of the gene is on the long arm of chromosome 22 at 22q13.1 (Fig. 4.1).

CYP2D6 consists of approximately 4,383 nucleotides. Given that 1,000 nucleotides are referred to as a kilobase, CYP2D6 can be described as being 4.4 kilobases in size. CYP2D6 contains nine exons that are composed of 1,491 nucleotides (Fig. 4.2). The CYP2D6 gene codes for the 2D6 enzyme, which is composed of 497 amino acids.

CYP2D6 is highly variable, and newly discovered rare variants are still being regularly identified. Each specific genetic variation that has been reported in the scientific literature is reviewed for authenticity at the Karolinska Institute in Stockholm. If a variant is demonstrated to be novel, the allele is catalogued on the institute website (http://www.cypalleles.ki.se/). Currently, there are 130 known variants, although only 75 formally recognized alleles have been given a "*" (i.e., star) designation. The other 55 variants have not been formally determined to be unique because they are very similar to other, previously designated

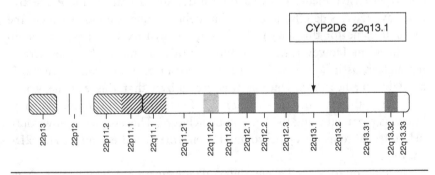

Figure 4.1. Chromosome 22 with arrow to designate the location of CYP2D6.

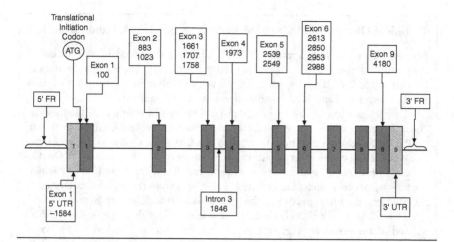

FIGURE 4.2. CYP2D6 structure illustrating the location of the nine exons and the 16 single nucleotide polymorphisms (SNPs) that define the most important CYP2D6 alleles. Each of these SNPs is designated by a number reflecting the nucleotide location of the SNP along the sequence of the gene.

* alleles. Clinical pharmacogenomic reports of CYP2D6 specify the two * alleles that define the genotype. For example, a patient with a *1/*4 genotype has one copy of the *1 allele and one copy of the *4 allele.

Table 4.1 lists the 16 CYP2D6 allele variations that are currently identified in most clinical reference laboratories and the activity level of the enzyme produced by each of these alleles.

TABLE 4.1. The activity level of 16 commonly genotyped CYP2D6 alleles

Allele	Activity Level	Northern European Allele Frequency (%)
*1	Normal	37
*2A	Increased	21
*2B	Decreased	<1
*2D	Decreased	<1
*3	None	2
*4	None	19
*5	None	3
*6	None	1
*7	None	<1
*8	None	<1
*9	Decreased	3
*10	Decreased	2
*11	None	<1
*15	None	<1
*17	Decreased	<1
*41	Decreased	9

Technical Discussion of CYP2D6 Variations (see Fig. 4.2 and Table 4.2)

Each of the most well-studied CYP2D6 alleles is described in this technical discussion. Although clinicians do not need to learn the precise nucleotide changes that influence CYP2D6 enzyme activity level, the following section is presented for those who are interested in molecular genetic mechanisms.

The designation of the *1 has been conventionally reserved to identify the "normal" form of the gene for all of the cytochrome P450 genes, including CYP2D6. Geneticists traditionally refer to this form of the gene as the *wild type*, and consider all of the other variations to be *mutants*. In the case of CYP2D6, the *1 allele produces an active form of the enzyme that is the "standard" by which the activity of other alleles is calibrated. Table 4.2 shows the specific variations of the gene and the locations of variable single nucleotide polymorphisms.

Two alleles of CYP2D6 have the same single nucleotide polymorphism (SNP) located in the promoter region. One of these variants is *2A, which has been reported to result in a somewhat enhanced production of normally active 2D6 enzyme. *2A has a cytosine to guanine change at the –1584 nucleotide location, which is in the promoter region, and a second SNP at nucleotide location 2850 in exon 6 that consists of a cytosine to thymine change. The second allele that has a guanine change at nucleotide location –1584 is *41, which produces an enzyme with decreased activity despite having the –1584 promoter variant.

In addition to *2A, 12 other *2 alleles are currently listed on the Karolinska website (http://www.cypalleles.ki.se/). They are designated as *2B through *2M. All of them have the common cytosine to thymine SNP at the 2850 nucleotide location in exon 6, which defines them all as members of the family of *2 alleles. All of these *2 alleles also have a guanine to cytosine change at the 4180 nucleotide location in exon 9 and most of these *2 alleles have a guanine-to-cytosine change at the 1661 nucleotide location in exon 3. However, each of these twelve *2 variants are further differentiated by additional SNPs. The activity level of the relatively rare alleles *2B and *2D has not been definitively established, but is probably somewhat decreased. Further clarification of activity levels of these alleles with different 2D6 substrates is still needed (Marez et al., 1997). An interesting "derivative allele" of the *2 family is the *41 allele. As noted previously, *41 has a cytosine to guanine change at nucleotide location –1584. *41 also has SNPs at nucleotide locations 2850 and 4180 that characterize all of the currently designated *2 alleles. However, as a consequence of the guanine-to-adenine change at location 2988 in exon 6, the enzyme produced by the *41 allele has decreased activity.

The *5 allele refers to the special situation that occurs when the entire CYP2D6 gene has been deleted from chromosome 22. Given that the gene is completely missing, *5 is only referred to as an "allele" by convention.

Three important alleles have been created by "small" deletions. The *3 allele has been created by the deletion of a single adenine at nucleotide location 2549 in exon 5. The *6 allele has been created by a single thymine deletion at nucleotide location 1707 in exon 3. The *9 allele has been created by a deletion of three nucleotides at positions 2613, 2614, and 2615 in exon 6. The *3 and *6 allele deletions each create a frame shift in the reading frame of the gene. Consequently, these two alleles produce a protein product that has no functional activity. In contrast, the *9 allele has been created by the loss of a complete codon consisting

(*continued on p. 36*)

TABLE 4.2. CYP2D6 variations that define 16 common alleles

CYP2D6 Allele	Enzyme Activity	5'UTR -1584	Exon 1 100	Exon 2 883	1023	1661	Exon 3 1707	1758	Intron 3 1846	Exon 4 1973	Exon 5 2539	2549	2613	Exon 6 2850	2935	2988	Exon 9 4180
*1	Normal	C	C	G	C	G	T	G	G	G	A	A	A	C	A	G	G
*2A	Increased	G	C	G	C	C	T	G	G	G	A	A	A	T	A	G	C
*2B	Decreased	C	C	G	C	C	T	G	G	G	A	A	A	T	A	G	C
*2D	Decreased	C	C	G	C	G	T	G	G	G	A	A	A	T	A	G	C
*3	None	C	C	G	C	G	T	G	G	G	A	DELETION of A in Exon 5 at 2549 Frame Shift to Left					
*4	None	C	T	G	C	C	T	G	A	G	A	A	A	C	A	G	C
*6	None	C	C	G	C	G	DELETION of T in Exon 3 at 1707 Frame Shift Left	G	G	G	A	A	A	C	C	G	G
*7	None	C	C	G	C	G	T	G	G	G	A	A	A	T	A	G	C
*8	None	C	C	G	C	C	T	T	G	G	A	A	A	C	A	G	G
*9	Decreased	C	C	G	C	G	T	G	G	G	A	A	Del AAG	C	A	G	G
*10	Decreased	C	T	G	C	C	T	G	G	G	A	A	A	C	A	G	C
*11	None	C	C	C	C	C	T	G	G	G	A	A	A	T	A	G	C
*12	None	C	C	G	C	C	T	G	G	G	A	A	A	T	A	G	C
*15	None	C	C	INSERTION of T in Exon 1 at 138 Frame Shift to Right													
*17	Decreased	C	C	G	T	C	T	G	G	G	A	A	A	T	A	G	C
*41	Decreased	G	C	G	C	C	T	G	G	G	A	A	A	T	A	A	C

This table documents the specific nucleotide variations that define the most common alleles of CYP2D6. Each row represents an allele, which is designated by a "*" and a number, except *2A, *2B, and *2D. Each column represents a location on the gene map. The *1 row is the "wild type" reference sequence that codes for a completely functional form of the CYP2D6 enzyme. The *2A, *2B, *2D, *3, *4, *6, *7, *8, *9, *10, *11, *12, *15, *17, and *41 are variations of the *1 wild type. The nucleotides that are shaded represent variations from the wild type reference sequence. Note that *5 is not included because a patient designated as having a *5 allele actually has a complete deletion of CYP2D6.

(*Continued*)

of three nucleotides. Given that there is no frame shift, the protein product of this allele has some preserved, although decreased, activity.

One important allele has been created because of an insertion. The *15 allele has been created by the insertion of a thymine between two nucleotides at locations 138 and 139 in exon 1. Since this insertion creates a frame shift change in the reading frame, the enzyme produced by *15 has no functional activity.

Six more alleles are the result of still other SNPs. Some of these alleles are very common in certain ethnic populations, and all of them result in either a decrease or a complete loss of enzyme activity. The *4 allele has 13 variations, designated *4A to *4M. All of these alleles have a common guanine to adenine change at nucleotide location 1846 in intron 3. This SNP results in a splicing defect, so that all *4 alleles produce a protein product that has no functional activity. The *7 allele results in an adenine to cytosine change at nucleotide location 2935 in exon 6, which also results in the production of an inactive protein product. The *8 allele has a guanine-to-thymine change at nucleotide location 1758 in exon 3, which produces a *stop codon*. Consequently, the *8 allele produces no functional protein product. The *10 allele has four variations, but all of them share a common cytosine to thymine change at nucleotide location 100 in exon 1. While this results in a folding problem in the structure of the 2D6 protein, the enzyme produced by the *10 allele does preserve some limited ability to metabolize 2D6 substrates. The *11 allele has a guanine to cytosine change at nucleotide location 883 in exon 2, which results in a splicing defect. Consequently, the *11 produces a protein product with no enzymatic activity. Finally, the *17 allele has a change from a cytosine to thymine at nucleotide location 1023 in exon 2, as well as the common cytosine to thymine change at nucleotide location 2850 in exon 6. These changes result in the *17 allele producing a protein product with some reduced functional activity.

GENOTYPIC VARIANCE ACROSS GEOGRAPHIC ANCESTRY

The population frequency of CYP2D6 alleles varies across racial and ethnic groups. The pattern of this CYP2D6 variability provides insights into the process of human evolution. It also highlights the clinical utility of using genotyping to guide pharmacological decisions in patient populations of different geographic ancestry. To illustrate this variation, five different population groups, all of which have been extensively studied, will be described and contrasted to highlight their substantial allelic variations. The populations reviewed come from various geographic regions of the world: Northern Europeans, Ethiopians, Sub-Saharan Africans, Japanese, and South American Indians. The overall estimates of the allele frequencies in these groups can be misleading (Table 4.3), as the precise frequencies of specific alleles can be quite different in small communities within these large geographic regions, because of variable migration, admixture, and prolonged isolation (Ingelman-Sundberg, 2005).

TABLE 4.3. Variability in key allele frequencies in five groups with different geographic ancestry

Geographic Ancestry	*1 (%)	*3 (%)	*4 (%)	*9 (%)	*10 (%)	*17 (%)	Active Duplications
Northern European	37	2	19	3	2	<0.1	2
Ethiopian	55	<0.1	3	<0.1	6	6	30
Sub-Saharan African	52	<0.1	2	<0.1	4	30	3
Japanese	48	<0.1	<0.1	<0.1	50	<0.1	Only *10Dup
South American Indians	73	<0.1	3	<0.1	1	<0.1	3

Northern Europeans

Northern Europeans have some alleles that are completely inactive and found in no other geographic ancestral group. For example, the CYP2D6*3 and CYP2D6*9 alleles occur almost exclusively in European populations. The CYP2D6*3 allele frequency occurs in only about 2% of Northern Europeans, whereas the CYP2D6*9 allele occurs in about 3% of Northern Europeans. However, the precise allele frequencies of these relatively rare alleles do vary considerably between different Northern European communities. The most common inactive allele in European populations is CYP2D6*4, which approaches a frequency of 20% in some communities. In contrast, the CYP2D6*17 allele very rarely occurs in Europeans, and the allele frequency of CYP2D6*10 is only 3%. The frequency of the ultra-rapid metabolizer phenotype, which is defined as having three or more copies of active CYP2D6 alleles, is only about 2% in Northern Europeans.

Ethiopians

In Ethiopia, about 30% of the population has CYP2D6 duplications of active alleles, as compared to a frequency of about 2% in Northern European populations. Ethiopians have a CYP2D6*4 allele frequency of 3%, and this is believed to reflect an admixture of European alleles that have been introduced into North Africa. However, virtually no individuals in Ethiopia have either the CYP2D6*3 or the CYP2D6*9 alleles. Finally, Ethiopians have a CYP2D6*17 allele frequency of 6%, which is much lower than the CYP2D6*17 allele frequency in Sub-Saharan Africans.

Sub-Saharan Africans

The allele frequency of CYP2D6*17 is about 30% in Sub-Saharan populations, whereas only 3% of the population carries chromosomes with duplications of active alleles. These allele frequencies are clearly different from Ethiopian allele frequencies. The allele frequency of CYP2D6*4 in Sub-Saharan Africa is only 2%, and there is virtually no incidence of CYP2D6*3 or CYP2D6*9 in Sub-Saharan Africans.

Japanese

The Japanese population has virtually no incidence of CYP2D6*3, CYP2D6*4, CYP2D6*9, or CYP2D6*17 alleles, reflecting its long isolation from European populations. However, the allele frequency of CYP2D6*10 is about 50%. The Japanese rarely have duplications of active CYP2D6 alleles, but they do have duplications of the CYP2D6*10 allele.

South American Indians

South American Indian populations have virtually no incidence of CYP2D6*3, CYP2D6*9, or CYP2D6*17 alleles. They have a CYP2D6*4 allele frequency of only 3% and a CYP2D6*10 allele frequency of 1%. They have a 3% frequency of active CYP2D6 duplications. However, other undefined variants of CYP2D6 may well exist in South American populations, because they have not been as extensively studied as other geographic ancestry groups.

Challenges in Characterizing Hispanic Populations

The development of an identity that is designated "Hispanic" is primarily the result of the establishment of a shared culture that includes speaking the Spanish language. However, major genetic variations occur across different geographic populations that identify themselves as Hispanic. The CYP2D6 allele frequencies in Spanish-speaking cultures reflect their quite different biological heritages. A Hispanic living in Spain will have allelic frequencies that are similar to Western European populations, with the exception of having a 10% frequency of duplications of active CYP2D6 alleles, which is believed to be a consequence of the Moorish migration into Spain from North Africa. A Hispanic living in the Caribbean will have a relatively high frequency of the CYP2D6*17 allele, reflecting African geographic ancestry. Finally, a Hispanic from the indigenous population of Mexico will have virtually no incidence of CYP2D6*17 and a very low incidence of CYP2D6*4 and CYP2D6*10, reflecting the allele distribution of the native South American population.

Hispanic patients drawn from all three geographic regions will include some individuals who are poor metabolizers and others who are ultra-rapid metabolizers. However, to accurately genotype these Hispanic patients from different geographic ancestral origins, it is necessary to test for quite different alleles. Once the correct genotype is established, the metabolic phenotype can be predicted without any knowledge of cultural identity.

Defining CYP2D6 Metabolic Phenotypes

Most individuals have two copies of CYP2D6, and their genotype is defined by these two alleles. Additionally, CYP2D6 can be deleted from one or both of the two copies of chromosomes 22 of an individual patient. This can result in an individual having a single copy of CYP2D6 on one of their chromosomes or no copy of CYP2D6 on either chromosome. It is not necessary to have a copy of CYP2D6 for survival, as patients with the *5/*5 genotype are missing CYP2D6 on both of their two 22nd chromosomes.

As has been reviewed, it is also possible to have two or more copies of CYP2D6 on a single chromosome. For example, a patient may have two copies of CYP2D6 on one of their 22nd chromosomes and one copy of CYP2D6 on the other, or a patient may have multiple copies of CYP2D6 on each chromosome. Thirteen copies of CYP2D6 have been reported to occur in one unusual patient (Dalen et al., 1998).

Given the large number of CYP2D6 alleles, thousands of possible CYP2D6 genotypes can result from the various possible pairings of variant alleles on the two chromosomes. However, by tradition, this enormous variability has been made more manageable by classifying patients into four broad clinical CYP2D6 metabolic phenotypes: 1) poor metabolizers, 2) intermediate metabolizers, 3) extensive or normal metabolizers, and 4) ultra-rapid metabolizers.

Considerable confusion has been generated in the literature because different methodologies have been used to determine these four phenotypes. For the sake of clarity, the two most common methods will be described as the "current" method and the "historical" method. The current method is the most commonly used in contemporary papers. The historical method was used frequently before 2000, and is still used to interpret the phenotypic results of the Amplichip, a common genotyping method that was approved by the U.S. Food and Drug Administration (FDA) in 2004. The current methodology classifies more patients as intermediate metabolizers, many of whom the historical method would label as extensive metabolizers. Consequently, the current method identifies more individuals as being potentially sensitive to medication and who may require lower doses of CYP2D6 substrate medications to minimize possible side effects.

An illustration of the importance of using the current method is demonstrated by genotyping subjects who participated in the Sequenced Treatment Alternatives to Relieve Depression study (Star*D), which is a large effectiveness trial of treatment using antidepressant medications. Using the current method, 40% of the sample would be classified as intermediate metabolizers. In contrast, using the historical method, only 4% of the Star*D sample would be classified as intermediate metabolizers. The remaining 36% of the sample would be categorized as extensive metabolizers, even though they have one inactive allele. The current method identifies more patients who are at some increased risk for side effects of 2D6 substrate medication and should be more closely monitored when using 2D6 substrate medications.

Furthermore, 3% of the subjects from the Star*D study, whom the historical method would classify as extensive metabolizers, would be classified by the current method as ultra-rapid. This change in classification would alert clinicians to possible problems related to subclinical response. One genotype, *2A/*2A, would identify patients as being extensive metabolizers using the historical model, but these patients actually have increased metabolic capacity and would be classified by the current method as being ultra-rapid metabolizers. The historical method does not consider the *2A allele to be sufficiently upregulated to treat patients who have two copies of the *2A allele as ultra-rapid metabolizers.

There are many possible pairings of deficient alleles and inactive alleles. Individuals with these pairings have significantly reduced enzyme activity and are classified by the current phenotyping method as poor metabolizers. However, when using the historical method, these patients would be classified as intermediate metabolizers.

Another genotype, which has changed in the interpretation of phenotypes, is found in individuals with an enhanced or a normal allele paired with an inactive allele. Individuals with these genotypes were classified by the historical method as being extensive metabolizers. However, they produce a less-functional enzyme and are more appropriately labeled as intermediate metabolizers, using the current phenotype method. The current method was used by Kirchheiner (2004) to identify specific dosage modification of many common psychotropic medications based on the derived phenotypes of patients.

Current Definition of the Poor Metabolizer Phenotype

Using the currently accepted methodology, a poor metabolizer is defined as an individual who has two completely inactive copies of CYP2D6 or one inactive and one deficient copy (Kirchheiner, 2004). This is in contrast to the historical classification system that restricted the definition of a poor metabolizer to an individual with two completely inactive alleles.

Current Definition of the Intermediate Metabolizer Phenotype

The current phenotyping methodology classifies individuals with one active copy and one inactive or deficient copy as intermediate metabolizers (Kirchheiner et al., 2004). Individuals with two deficient copies are usually categorized as intermediate, despite the fact that some pairs of deficient alleles will result in quite poor metabolism of some 2D6 substrates and more effective metabolism of other 2D6 substrates. The historical methodology restricted the classification of an intermediate metabolizer to those individuals who have one totally inactive copy and one partially active or deficient copy.

The most obvious problem that arises when using the historical methodology is that an individual who has one active and one inactive allele is categorized as being an extensive metabolizer. However, pharmacokinetic studies have demonstrated that individuals with one active and one inactive or deficient allele have higher serum levels of CYP2D6 substrate medications at any given therapeutic dose when compared to individuals with two active copies (Dalen et al., 1998). Individuals with one inactive copy and one inactive or deficient copy have also been reported to have had an increased incidence of side effects when taking CYP2D6 substrate medications (McAlpine et al., 2007).

Current Definition of the Extensive Metabolizer Phenotype

In current practice, the phenotype of an "extensive" metabolizer is reserved for individuals with two fully active copies or one active and one enhanced allele of CYP2D6. The historical methodology would additionally classify individuals with one active and one inactive allele as being extensive metabolizers.

Current Definition of the Ultra-rapid Metabolizer Phenotype

Ultra-rapid CYP2D6 metabolizers are usually defined as individuals who have three or more active copies of CYP2D6. However, individuals who are homozygous for enhanced CYP2D6 alleles that contain the −1584 promoter variant (e.g., *2A) are also able to produce more enzyme than those who are homozygous for the *1 allele, although they produce less enzyme than an individual with three active copies of CYP2D6. An additional classification challenge is encountered in an individual who has two active copies of the gene and one partially active copy. While no uniformly accepted convention has been established to phenotype these patients, they would be expected to produce more 2D6 enzyme than a patient with only two active alleles and therefore have relatively more rapid metabolism. A conservative approach to phenotyping is to classify all patients with increased production of 2D6 enzyme in the ultra-rapid category.

A Seven-category Phenotyping Strategy

A seven-category classification system has also been adopted by some laboratories, instead of the traditional four phenotypic categories. By creating three

TABLE 4.4. Comparison of the traditional phenotypes and the seven-category phenotypes

Traditional Phenotypes	Seven-category Phenotypes	Definition of Seven-category Phenotypes
Ultra-rapid	Ultra-rapid	• >2 alleles with normal activity or • ≥2 alleles with increased activity
Extensive	Enhanced extensive	• 1 allele with increased activity and 1 allele with normal activity
	Extensive	• 2 normal activity alleles or • 1 allele with increased activity and 1 allele with decreased activity
Intermediate	Enhanced intermediate	• 1 increased activity allele paired with an allele with no activity or • 1 normal activity allele paired with an allele with decreased activity or • 3 alleles with decreased activity
	Intermediate	• 1 normal activity allele paired with an allele with no activity or • 2 alleles with decreased activity
Poor	Reduced intermediate	• 1 allele with decreased activity paired with 1 allele with no activity
	Poor	• No alleles with any level of activity

new phenotypic categories, the seven-category strategy can identify more homogenous groups of patients. These new categories have been labeled as the *enhanced extensive phenotype*, the *enhanced intermediate phenotype*, and the *reduced intermediate phenotype* (Table 4.4).

While the seven-category genotype classification is a more precise method for grouping patients into phenotypic categories based on metabolic capacity, the current clinical literature primarily describes patients who have been classified into the four traditional phenotypes. Unfortunately, very old literature includes a number of idiosyncratic methodologies for phenotypically classifying patients. For example, in some of the earliest papers, patients were simply assigned to one of two categories: poor and not poor. In the future, it seems probable that more refined phenotyping methodologies such as the seven-category solution, will be utilized in clinical research studies and clinical practice.

CYP2D6 PHENOCOPIES

A *phenocopy* refers to the identification of a phenotypic characteristic in an individual that is the result of an environmental factor rather than a genetic variation. This characteristic may be quite similar to a phenotype that is the result of gene expression.

A pharmacogenomic CYP2D6 phenocopy occurs when an environmental factor influences gene expression or enzyme function, resulting in patients who metabolize 2D6 medications in a different manner than would be predicted by their genotype. This occurs regularly because of drug–drug interactions. An important clinical example is the use of medications that are strong inhibitors of the 2D6 enzyme. However, the degree to which 2D6 inhibition occurs in patients with different CYP2D6 genotypes has not been completely demonstrated. Some controversy emerged over this issue when consideration of data derived from two quite different sources arrived at different conclusions. The first source of data is from the analysis of pharmacokinetic studies that are usually limited to a small cohort of patients. These reports are usually based on a limited number of observations, but they have the appearance of being scientifically rigorous because the precise serum levels of 2D6 substrate medications can be accurately and reliably measured and reported. The second source of data is derived from clinical practice, where a very large number of clinical observations can be made over the course of many years. Clinical conclusions that are drawn from a large series of observations have been categorized as being subjective or "anecdotal." However, they may also be correct.

The most common poor CYP2D6 phenocopy is found in a patient who does not have a poor CYP2D6 genotype, but responds to 2D6 substrate medications as if he was a poor metabolizer. This can occur because of 2D6 enzyme inhibition. Fluoxetine and paroxetine are two selective serotonin reuptake inhibitors (SSRIs) that are quite effective 2D6 enzyme inhibitors. Paroxetine is of particular interest because it is almost exclusively metabolized by the 2D6 enzyme. Bupropion is another antidepressant that is also a potent inhibitor of CYP2D6 (Kotlyar et al., 2005).

To better illustrate the concept of a phenocopy, the effect of enzyme inhibition on individuals with each of the four major traditional phenotypes will be reviewed. An important concept to understand is that it is not possible to create a poor CYP2D6 phenocopy in a patient who produces no active enzyme as a consequence of having two inactive CYP2D6 alleles. Essentially, if the patient produces no active enzyme, it is not possible to further decrease his enzyme activity through enzyme inhibition.

Enzyme inhibition is particularly important in patients who have an intermediate 2D6 metabolism. Pharmacokinetic studies have shown that even moderate doses of fluoxetine or paroxetine in patients with an intermediate CYP2D6 phenotype can result in a change in their pharmacokinetic clearance of 2D6 substrate medications. Consequently, these patients develop high serum levels of medication that resembles the pharmacokinetic clearance of patients who are poor metabolizers based on their genotype (Preskorn, 2003).

Patients with two active copies of CYP2D6 may also be converted into de facto poor metabolizers when given an enzyme inhibitor, as pharmacokinetic studies of such patients have demonstrated higher serum levels of prescribed 2D6 substrate medications after enzyme inhibition. However, the results of these studies must be reconciled with what is observed in clinical practice, where many patients who are extensive metabolizers are maintained on the recommended doses of fluoxetine and paroxetine without developing the adverse reactions that would be predicted by inhibition of the 2D6 enzyme.

Ultra-rapid metabolizers make an increased quantity of the 2D6 enzyme. They can take relatively high doses of fluoxetine or paroxetine and still not develop adverse reactions. Although this phenomenon has not been studied extensively, it is conceptually possible that inhibition will actually facilitate these patients in achieving a therapeutic blood level of 2D6 substrate medications. Further research is needed to be able to estimate the appropriate doses of fluoxetine and paroxetine in patients who are genetically ultra-rapid CYP2D6 metabolizers. However, in the absence of additional research, it is prudent to avoid prescribing 2D6 substrate medications for patients who have ultra-rapid 2D6 metabolism.

ANTIDEPRESSANT MEDICATIONS

A number of antidepressants are metabolized, primarily or partially, by the 2D6 enzyme (Table 4.5). Specifically, desipramine, doxepin, fluoxetine, nortriptyline, paroxetine, and venlafaxine are metabolized primarily by the 2D6 enzyme (Shimoda et al., 2000; Spina et al., 1997). One component of the designation that a substrate is "primarily" metabolized by the 2D6 enzyme is that no other CYP enzyme would normally be involved in its metabolism if an adequate concentration of a 2D6 enzyme were present. In contrast, amitriptyline, bupropion, duloxetine, imipramine, mirtazapine, and trazodone have substantial, but not exclusive, 2D6 substrate metabolic clearance (Skinner et al., 2003). The designation that the substrate is

TABLE 4.5. Antidepressant medications metabolized by the 2D6 enzyme

Antidepressants Primarily Metabolized by 2D6	Antidepressants Substantially Metabolized by 2D6	Antidepressants Minimally Metabolized by 2D6
Desipramine	Amitriptyline	Citalopram
Doxepin	Bupropion	Escitalopram
Fluoxetine	Duloxetine	Fluvoxamine
Nortriptyline	Imipramine	Sertraline
Paroxetine	Mirtazapine	
Venlafaxine	Trazodone	

"substantially" but not exclusively a 2D6 substrate refers to the fact that other CYP enzymes are normally involved in the metabolism of the substrate, even when an adequate amount of 2D6 enzyme is present.

The antidepressant bupropion presents an interesting pharmacogenetic challenge for patients with poor 2D6 metabolism. The cytochrome P450 2B6 enzyme is primarily responsible for the metabolism of bupropion to hydroxybupropion. However, hydroxybupropion is primarily metabolized by the 2D6 enzyme. Consequently, patients with no 2D6 activity may accumulate a high serum concentration of hydroxybupropion. This elevated serum level of hydroxybupropion may be a mechanism that contributes to some of the more severe adverse reactions to bupropion, such as seizures.

The 2D6 enzyme plays a relatively minor role in the metabolic clearance of citalopram, escitalopram, fluvoxamine, and sertraline. However, the 2D6 enzyme provides a secondary metabolic pathway for all of these drugs, which can be important if their primary metabolic enzymes are not functional.

ANTIPSYCHOTIC MEDICATIONS

A number of antipsychotic medications are predominantly or partially metabolized by the 2D6 enzyme (Table 4.6) (Brockmoller et al., 2002; Dahl, 2002; Kudo & Ishizaki, 1999; Linnet & Olesen, 1997; Olesen & Linnet, 2000; Spina et al., 2003; Wojcikowski et al., 2006; Yoshii et al., 2000).

Risperidone is an atypical antipsychotic medication that is primarily metabolized by the 2D6 enzyme, and poor CYP2D6 metabolizers have been shown to have an increased frequency of side effects when taking standard doses of this medication (de Leon et al., 2005). Patients who are poor metabolizers of 2D6 substrate medications have also been shown to have an increased probability for hyperprolactinemia, because of accumulation of 9-hydroxyrisperidone, when prescribed risperidone. The metabolite, 9-hydroxyrisperidone, is one of the first metabolites of risperidone (Spina et al., 2001). Individuals who are ultra-rapid metabolizers of 2D6 substrate medication are unlikely to achieve adequate serum levels when taking standard doses of risperidone.

TABLE 4.6. Antipsychotic medications metabolized by the 2D6 enzyme

Antipsychotic Medications Primarily Metabolized by 2D6	Antipsychotic Medications Substantially Metabolized by 2D6	Antipsychotic Medications Minimally Metabolized by 2D6
Chlorpromazine	Aripiprazole	Clozapine
Haloperidol	Olanzapine	Quetiapine
Perphenazine		Ziprasidone
Risperidone		
Thioridazine		

Aripiprazole is another atypical antipsychotic medication metabolized by the 2D6 enzyme. However, since aripiprazole is also metabolized by the 3A4 enzyme, it is usually possible for CYP2D6 poor-metabolizing patients to tolerate aripiprazole at reduced doses.

Four of the typical antipsychotic medications are predominantly metabolized by the 2D6 enzyme. Two of these medications, chlorpromazine and thioridazine, are now rarely used because of their side-effect profiles. However, haloperidol is still a widely utilized typical antipsychotic medication despite a high occurrence of extrapyramidal side effects. Perphenazine is also still in use and has been shown to have comparable efficacy to the most widely used atypical antipsychotics (Lieberman et al., 2005). Additional research is needed to clarify how CYP2D6 genotypic variations that predict the poor metabolizer phenotype may be related to the development of specific adverse side effects.

OTHER MEDICATIONS THAT ARE 2D6 SUBSTRATES

Atomoxetine

Atomoxetine is a 2D6 substrate medication used to treat patients with attention-deficit hyperactivity disorder. Poor CYP2D6 metabolizers develop high serum levels of atomoxetine that can lead to adverse reactions, including severe sedation. However, poor CYP2D6 metabolizers who are able to tolerate atomoxetine may have a positive therapeutic response, which may be mediated by sustaining higher serum levels (Michelson et al., 2007).

Codeine

Codeine is a pro-drug, which means that it is not pharmacologically active and must be metabolized to achieve a therapeutic response. Essentially, a patient requires adequate 2D6 enzyme activity to metabolize codeine to morphine in order to achieve effective analgesia. Consequently, individuals who have the poor 2D6 metabolizer phenotype do not experience adequate pain relief when taking codeine. In contrast, ultra-rapid metabolizers experience a rapid surge of morphine after they take an oral dose of codeine that can be experienced as either euphoric or dysphoric.

A specific indication exists for CYP2D6 genotyping in young mothers who are given codeine for postpartum analgesia. Since ultra-rapid metabolizers rapidly convert codeine to morphine, a high dose of morphine can be transferred to the infant of a mother who is an ultra-rapid metabolizer and is breast-feeding. Even relatively modest doses of codeine taken by a breast-feeding mother who is an ultra-rapid metabolizer can result in a toxic level of morphine in her infant, as demonstrated by the death of a 13-day-old breast-fed infant whose mother was an ultra-rapid metabolizer. The fatal reaction of this infant to the morphine in the breast milk of his mother occurred when she was being prescribed modest doses of acetaminophen with codeine for her episiotomy pain (Koren et al., 2006).

Tramadol

Tramadol is an analgesic and, like codeine, a pro-drug. Inadequate analgesia with tramadol is experienced in patients who are poor metabolizers of 2D6 substrate medications. Additionally, the abuse potential of tramadol may be greater in patients who are ultra-rapid metabolizers of 2D6 substrate medications.

Dextromethorphan

Dextromethorphan is a 2D6 substrate medication commonly used as a cough suppressant, and it is contained in many over-the-counter cold preparations (e.g., Nyquil and Robitussin-DM). High doses of dextromethorphan can provide a sense of altered awareness in patients who are poor 2D6 metabolizers and can increase the risk of abuse. Individuals with the poor metabolizer phenotype can build up elevated serum levels of dextromethorphan more rapidly than can extensive metabolizers. In contrast, ultra-rapid CYP2D6 metabolizers, who quickly metabolize dextromethorphan, are at low risk of abusing this medication and are unlikely to derive antitussive benefit at traditional doses.

Ectasy or 3,4-Methylenedioxy-N-methylamphetamine (MDMA)

MDMA (3,4-methylenedioxy-N-methylamphetamine) or Ecstasy is a semi-synthetic member of the amphetamine class of psychoactive drugs. MDMA is demethylenated by the 2D6 enzyme. A study of MDMA metabolism has shown that the CYP2D6*17 and the CYP2D6 *10 alleles produce forms of the CYP2D6 enzyme that display substrate-specific changes in drug affinity. Specifically, individuals who have the CYP2D6*17 or CYP2D6*10 alleles were less able to effectively metabolize MDMA and were at greater risk of toxicity (Ramamoorthy et al., 2002).

Tamoxifen

Tamoxifen is an orally active selective estrogen receptor modulator that is the most widely prescribed medication for the treatment of breast cancer. Tamoxifen is a pro-drug that requires adequate 2D6 metabolism to achieve a therapeutic response. The 2D6 enzyme facilitates the metabolism of tamoxifen to endoxifen, which is the active form of this medication. Women who have poor 2D6 metabolic activity are unable to benefit fully from the therapeutic effects of tamoxifen (Goetz et al., 2007; Goetz et al., 2005; Jin et al., 2005). Consequently, CYP2D6 genotyping is indicated before prescribing tamoxifen. Tamoxifen metabolism also can be affected by 2D6 enzyme–inhibiting drugs such as paroxetine, which blocks the metabolism of tamoxifen to endoxifen. Patients who are intermediate CYP2D6 metabolizers are particularly vulnerable to inhibition of the CYP2D6 enzyme.

CLINICAL IMPLICATIONS

The current clinical applications of CYP2D6 genotyping are straightforward. Essentially, patients with the poor 2D6 metabolizer phenotype require either the prescription of a medication that is not a 2D6 substrate or a reduced dosage of a 2D6 substrate medication. Intermediate 2D6 metabolizers require a modest decrease from the standard dose of a 2D6 substrate medication. Extensive or normal 2D6 metabolizers may be prescribed 2D6 substrate medications as directed. Finally, ultra-rapid CYP2D6 metabolizers will clear 2D6 substrate medications from the serum very quickly. Consequently, these medications should not generally be selected for these patients. While an alternative strategy might be to provide increased doses of 2D6 substrate medications to patients who are ultra-rapid metabolizers, with the goal of achieving therapeutic serum levels, this strategy requires close monitoring of the patient because intermediate metabolites may accumulate and lead to adverse and potentially dangerous effects.

The use of pharmacogenetic genotyping of CYP2D6 has become standard practice in many medical settings. The potential benefits of using CYP2D6 genotyping in the management of depression with antidepressant medications have been known for many years (Kirchheiner et al., 2001; Weinshilboum, 2003). However, some researchers have questioned the extent of these benefits in patients without psychotic symptoms who are being treated with SSRIs (Berg et al., 2007).

The clearest indication for CYP2D6 testing is to avoid adverse reactions by identifying patients who are poor metabolizers of 2D6 substrate medications. Extreme cases have been reported of patients who have died as a consequence of toxicity with fluoxetine (Sallee, DeVane, & Ferrell, 2000) and doxepin (Koski et al., 2007). While lethal iatrogenic deaths are fortunately relatively rare, an increase in side effects in patients who have the poor

CYP2D6 metabolizer phenotype is common and occurs with both antidepressants and antipsychotics.

Two additional considerations further justify the identification of patients with the poor metabolizer phenotype when using SSRIs that are 2D6 substrate medications. The first is that such patients may be more likely to develop suicidal ideation during the first weeks of treatment with 2D6 substrate antidepressant medications because of a rapid rise in serum level of these medications. The second consideration is that patients with the poor CYP2D6 metabolizer phenotype who have a genetic vulnerability to develop bipolar disorder may be more likely to have an activation of a manic episode if treated with an SSRI that is a 2D6 substrate medication at standard doses. The precise determination of the frequency of these adverse events will require further research, but these side effects are commonly reported and may be avoidable through more appropriate medication selection and dosing.

The identification of ultra-rapid CYP2D6 metabolizers may ultimately prove to be an even more important indication for CYP2D6 genotyping. It has been well established that patients with the ultra-rapid CYP2D6 metabolizer phenotype do not benefit from the use of 2D6 substrate medications at standard doses. While this may affect only 1 in 50 individuals of European ancestry, this absence of clinical benefit may occur in as many as 3 of every 10 patients who are of Northeast African origin. Without genotyping, it may take years to realize that a patient has an ultra-rapid metabolizer phenotype and will not benefit from treatment with 2D6 substrate medications at standard doses.

Clinical Case 1

A 16-year-old boy was doing well in high school and was generally well adjusted until he became ill with a severe upper respiratory infection. He was treated with large doses of an over-the-counter cold preparation. After taking a second large dose in a 4-hour interval, the patient became disoriented, confused, and had difficulty walking. His symptoms were attributed to his being quite ill with his respiratory illness. Over the course of 2 days, he began to express suicidal ideation for the first time in his life and composed a suicide note. He subsequently took eight ibuprofen tablets and confessed to his parents that he had taken an overdose. His parents took him to the emergency room where he was evaluated. Based on his having taken an overdose and having written a suicide note, it was determined that he was depressed. He was prescribed a 10 mg dose of fluoxetine. Within a week, he had no depressive symptoms.

The parents subsequently brought him to see a psychiatrist at an academic medical center for a second opinion. His CYP2D6 genotype revealed that he was a poor CYP2D6 metabolizer (Table 4.7).

(*Continued*)

TABLE 4.7. Pharmacogenomic report of case 1

Pharmacogenomic Report of Case 1		
Gene	Genotype of Patient	Clinical Implication
CYP2D6	*4/*4	Poor CYP2D6 metabolizer

In reviewing the history, it became clear that the patient had suffered from an adverse reaction to two large doses of dextromethorphan. His "depressive" symptoms resolved completely over the week following his overdose. His fluoxetine was consequently discontinued, as it was determined that he did not have a depressive illness. The patient finished the remainder of the school year with no recurrence of any psychiatric symptoms.

KEY CLINICAL CONSIDERATIONS

For patients with the CYP2D6 *poor metabolizer phenotype:*

- Avoid using 2D6 substrate medication at recommended doses.
- Avoid using dextromethorphan, as atypical psychiatric symptoms may occur with high serum levels.

For patients with the CYP2D6 *intermediate metabolizer phenotype:*

- Use 2D6 substrate medications at lower than the normally recommended doses.
- Do not prescribe medications that inhibit the 2D6 enzyme when prescribing psychotropic medications that are 2D6 substrates.

For patients with the CYP2D6 *ultra-rapid metabolizer phenotype:*

- Do not use 2D6 substrate medication at recommended doses. These medications should only be used at increased doses, if it is feasible to carefully monitor the patient to identify adverse reactions that may result as a consequence of high levels of secondary metabolites.

REFERENCES

Berg, A. O., Piper, M., Armstrong, K., Botkin, J., Calonge, N., Haddow, J., et al. (2007). Recommendations from the EGAPP Working Group: testing for cytochrome P450 polymorphisms in adults with nonpsychotic depression treated with selective serotonin reuptake inhibitors. *Genetics in Medicine: Official Journal of the American College of Medical Genetics, 9*(12), 819–825.

Brockmoller, J., Kirchheiner, J., Schmider, J., Walter, S., Sachse, C., Muller-Oerlinghausen, B., & Roots, I. (2002). The impact of the CYP2D6 polymorphism on haloperidol pharmacokinetics and on the outcome of haloperidol treatment. *Clinical Pharmacology and Therapeutics, 72,* 438–452

Dahl, M. L. (2002). Cytochrome p450 phenotyping/genotyping in patients receiving antipsychotics: useful aid to prescribing. *Clinical Pharmacokinetics, 41*(7), 453–470.

Dalen, P., Dahl, M. L., Ruiz, M. L., Nordin, J., & Bertilsson, L. (1998). 10-Hydroxylation of nortriptyline in white persons with 0, 1, 2, 3, and 13 functional CYP2D6 genes. *Clinical Pharmacology and Therapeutics 63*(4), 444–452.

Dayer, P., Kronbach, T., Eichelbaum, M., & Meyer, U. A. (1987). Enzymatic basis of the debrisoquine/sparteine-type genetic polymorphism of drug oxidation. Characterization of bufuralol 1'-hydroxylation in liver microsomes of in vivo phenotyped carriers of the genetic deficiency. *Biochemical Pharmacology, 36*(23), 4145–4152.

de Leon, J., Susce, M. T., Pan, R. M., Fairchild, M., Koch, W. H., & Wedlund, P. J. (2005). The CYP2D6 poor metabolizer phenotype may be associated with risperidone adverse drug reactions and discontinuation. *Journal of Clinical Psychiatry, 66*(1), 15–27.

Goetz, M. P., Knox, S. K., Suman, V. J., Rae, J. M., Safgren, S. L., Ames, M. M., et al. (2007). The impact of cytochrome P450 2D6 metabolism in women receiving adjuvant tamoxifen. *Breast Cancer Research and Treatment, 101*(1), 113–121.

Goetz, M. P., Rae, J. M., Suman, V. J., Safgren, S. L., Ames, M. M., Visscher, D. W., et al. (2005). Pharmacogenetics of tamoxifen biotransformation is associated with clinical outcomes of efficacy and hot flashes. *Journal of Clinical Oncology, 23*(36), 9312–9318.

Ingelman-Sundberg, M. (2005). Genetic polymorphisms of cytochrome P450 2D6 (CYP2D6): clinical consequences, evolutionary aspects and functional diversity. *Pharmacogenomics Journal, 5*(1), 6–13.

Jin, Y., Desta, Z., Stearns, V., Ward, B., Ho, H., Lee, K. H., et al. (2005). CYP2D6 genotype, antidepressant use, and tamoxifen metabolism during adjuvant breast cancer treatment. *Journal of the National Cancer Institute, 97*(1), 30–39.

Kimura, S., Umeno, M., Skoda, R., Meyer, U., & Gonzalez, F. (1989). The human debrisoquine 4-hydroxylase (CYP2D) locus: sequence and identification of the polymorphic CYP2D6 gene, a related gene, and a pseudogene. *American Journal of Human Genetics, 45*(6), 889–904.

Kirchheiner, J., Brosen, K., Dahl, M. L., Gram, L. F., Kasper, S., Roots, I., et al. (2001). CYP2D6 and CYP2C19 genotype-based dose recommendations for antidepressants: a first step towards subpopulation-specific dosages. *Acta Psychiatrica Scandinavica, 104*(3), 173–192.

Kirchheiner, J., Heesch, C., Bauer, S., Meisel, C., Seringer, A., Goldammer, M., et al. (2004). Impact of the ultrarapid metabolizer genotype of cytochrome

P450 2D6 on metoprolol pharmacokinetics and pharmacodynamics. *Clinical Pharmacology and Therapeutics, 76,* 302–312.

Kirchheiner, J., Nickchen, K., Bauer, M., Wong, M.-L., Licinio, J., Roots, I., & Brockmoller, J. (2004). Pharmacogenetics of antidepressants and antipsychotics: the contribution of allelic variations to the phenotype of drug response. *Molecular Psychiatry, 9,* 442–473.

Koren, G., Cairns, J., Chitayat, D., Gaedigk, A., & Leeder, S. J. (2006). Pharmacogenetics of morphine poisoning in a breastfed neonate of a codeine-prescribed mother. *Lancet, 368*(9536), 704.

Koski, A., Ojanpera, I., Vuori, E., & Sajantila, A. (2007). A fatal doxepin poisoning associated with a defective CYP2D6 genotype. *The American Journal of Forensic Medicine and Pathology, 28*(2):259–261.

Kotlyar, M., Brauer, L. H., Tracy, T. S., Hatsukami, D. K., Harris, J., Bronars, C. A., & Adson, D. E. (2005). Inhibition of CYP2D6 activity by bupropion. *Journal of Clinical Psychopharmacology, 25*(3), 226–229.

Kudo, S., & Ishizaki, T. (1999). Pharmacokinetics of haloperidol. *Clinical Pharmacokinetics, 37*(6), 435–456.

Lieberman, J. A., Stroup, T. S., McEvoy, J. P., Swartz, M. S., Rosenheck, R. A., Perkins, D. O., et al., CATIE Investigators. (2005). Effectiveness of antipsychotic drugs in patients with chronic schizophrenia. *New England Journal of Medicine, 353*(12), 1209–1223.

Linnet, K., & Olesen, O. V. (1997). Metabolism of clozapine by cDNA-expressed human cytochrome P450 enzymes. *Drug Metabolism & Disposition, 25*(12), 1379–1382.

Marez, D., Legrand, M., Sabbagh, N., Lo-Guidice, J., Lafitte, J., Meyer, U. A., & Broly, F. (1997). Polymorphism of the cytochrome P450 CYP2D6 gene in a European population: characterization of 48 mutations and 53 alleles, their frequencies and evolution. *Pharmacogenetics, 7,* 193–202.

McAlpine, D. E., O'Kane, D. J., Black, J. L., & Mrazek, D. A. (2007). Cytochrome P450 2D6 genotype variation and venlafaxine dosage. *Mayo Clinic Proceedings, 82*(9), 1065–1068.

Michelson, D., Read, H. A., Ruff, D. D., Witcher, J., Zhang, S., & McCracken, J. (2007). CYP2D6 and clinical response to atomoxetine in children and adolescents with ADHD. *Journal of the American Academy of Child & Adolescent Psychiatry, 46*(2), 242–251.

Olesen, O. V., & Linnet, K. (2000). Identification of the human cytochrome P450 isoforms mediating in vitro N-dealkylation of perphenazine. *British Journal of Clinical Pharmacology, 50*(6), 563–571.

Preskorn, S. (2003). Reproducibility of the in vivo effect of the selective serotonin reuptake inhibitors on the in vivo function of cytochrome P450 2D6: An update (part II). *Journal of Psychiatric Practice, 9*(2), 150–158.

Ramamoorthy, Y., Yu, A. M., Suh, N., Haining, R. L., Tyndale, R. F., & Sellers, E. M. (2002). Reduced (+/-)-3,4-methylenedioxymethamphetamine ("Ecstasy") metabolism with cytochrome P450 2D6 inhibitors and pharmacogenetic variants in vitro. *Biochemical Pharmacology, 63*(12), 2111–2119.

Sallee, F. R., DeVane, C. L., & Ferrell, R. E. (2000). Fluoxetine-related death in a child with cytochrome P-450 2D6 genetic deficiency. *Journal of Child & Adolescent Psychopharmacology, 10*(1), 27–34.

Shimoda, K., Morita, S., Hirokane, G., Yokono, A., Someya, T., & Takahashi, S. (2000). Metabolism of desipramine in Japanese psychiatric patients: The Impact of CYP2D6 genotyping on the hydroxylation of desipramine. *Pharmacoglogy & Toxicology, 86*, 245–249.

Skinner, M. H., Kuan, H. Y., Pan, A., Sathirakul, K., Knadler, M. P., Gonzales, C. R., et al. (2003). Duloxetine is both an inhibitor and a substrate of cytochrome P4502D6 in healthy volunteers. *Clinical Pharmacology and Therapeutics, 73*(3), 170–177.

Spina, E., Avenoso, A., Facciola, G., Salemi, M., Scordo, M. G., Ancione, M., et al. (2001). Relationship between plasma risperidone and 9-hydroxyrisperidone concentrations and clinical response in patients with schizophrenia. *Psychopharmacology, 153*(2), 238–243.

Spina, E., Gitto, C., Avenoso, A., Campo, G., Caputi, A., & Perucca, E. (1997). Relationship between plasma desipramine levels, CYP2D6 phenotype and clinical response to desipramine: a prospective study. *European Journal of Clinical Pharmacology, 51*, 395–398.

Spina, E., Scordo, M. G., & D'Arrigo, C. (2003). Metabolic drug interactions with new psychotropic agents. *Fundamental & Clinical Pharmacology, 17*(5), 517–538.

Weinshilboum, R. (2003). Inheritance and drug response. *New England Journal of Medicine, 348*(6), 529–537.

Wojcikowski, J., Maurel, P., & Daniel, W. A. (2006). Characterization of human cytochrome p450 enzymes involved in the metabolism of the piperidine-type phenothiazine neuroleptic thioridazine. *Drug Metabolism & Disposition, 34*(3), 471–476.

Yoshii, K., Kobayashi, K., Tsumuji, M., Tani, M., Shimada, N., & Chiba, K. (2000). Identification of human cytochrome P450 isoforms involved in the 7-hydroxylation of chlorpromazine by human liver microsomes. *Life Sciences, 67*(2), 175–184.

WEBSITES

Karolinska Institute: Human Cytochrome P450 (CYP) Allele Nomenclature Committee   http://www.cypalleles.ki.se/

5

THE CYTOCHROME P450 2C19 GENE

The cytochrome P450 2C19 gene (CYP2C19) was originally described as the mephenytoin hydroxylase gene (Kupfer et al., 1979). The original name was chosen because the enzyme produced by this gene has been demonstrated to be necessary for the hydroxylation of mephenytoin. Mephenytoin is an antiepileptic medication that is no longer widely used in clinical practice (Goldstein & de Morais, 1994; Wrighton et al., 1993). Consequently, the original name for this enzyme, mephenytoin hydroxylase, has become an anachronism. Like the CYP2D6 enzyme, the CYP2C19 enzyme is a member of the P450 family of enzymes. Consequently, mephenytoin hydroxylase has been renamed using the P450 nomenclature. This enzyme is now routinely referred to as the cytochrome 2C19 enzyme or simply the 2C19 enzyme.

Currently, over 50 available medications are primarily metabolized by the 2C19 enzyme. The 2C19 substrate medications include some quite commonly prescribed psychotropic medications. The 2C19 enzyme also plays a secondary role in the metabolism of many other drugs when their primary pathways are not functional. The genotyping of CYP2C19 is now widely available to clinicians.

LOCATION AND GENE VARIATION

CYP2C19 is located on chromosome 10, which is a much larger chromosome than chromosome 22, on which CYP2D6 is located. The specific location of the gene is on the long arm of chromosome 10 at 10q24.1-q24.3 (Fig. 5.1).

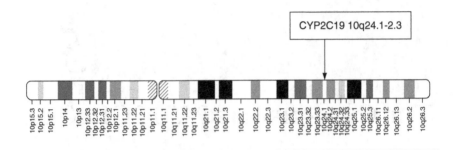

FIGURE 5.1. Chromosome 10 with arrow to designate the location of CYP2C19.

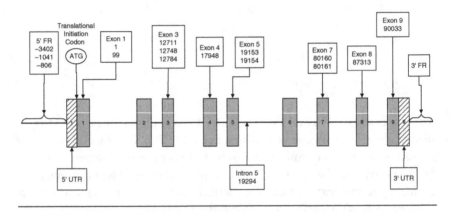

FIGURE 5.2. CYP2C19 structure illustrating the location of the nine exons and the 16 single nucleotide polymorphisms (SNPs) that define the most important CYP2C19 alleles. Each of these SNPs is designated by nucleotide location of the SNP along the sequence of the gene.

CYP2C19 is a relatively large gene, consisting of 90,209 nucleotides or 90.2 kilobases. It is approximately 30 times bigger than CYP2D6. However, like CYP2D6, CYP2C19 contains nine exons, which are composed of 1,473 nucleotides (Fig. 5.2). CYP2C19 codes for the CYP2C19 enzyme, which is composed of 490 amino acids and is seven amino acids smaller than the CYP2D6 enzyme.

Like CYP2D6, CYP2C19 is a highly variable gene, and newly identified rare variants are regularly discovered. The Karolinska Institute catalogues all of the variants on the institute's website (http://www.cypalleles.ki.se/). Currently, there are 31 known variants, although only 21 alleles have been given an official * (i.e., star) designation. The other ten variants have not been formally determined to be unique because they are very similar to other previously designated * (i.e., star) alleles.

TABLE 5.1. Activity level of eleven commonly genotyped CYP2C19 alleles

CYP2C19 Allele	Activity Level	Northern European Allele Frequency (%)
*1A, *1B, *1C	Normal	67
*2	None	14
*3	None	0.1
*4	None	<0.1
*5	None	<0.1
*6	None	<0.1
*7	None	<0.1
*8	None	<0.1
*9	Decreased	<0.1
*10	Decreased	<0.1
*17	Increased	18

Table 5.1 lists the 11 CYP2C19 variations currently identified in clinical reference laboratories and the activity level of the enzymes produced by these alleles. The frequency of each of these alleles in Northern European populations is also included in Table 5.1.

Technical Discussion of CYP2C19 Variations (see Fig. 5.2 and Table 5.2)

Each of the most well-studied CYP2C19 alleles is described in this technical discussion. Although clinicians do not need to learn the precise nucleotide changes that influence CYP2C19 enzyme activity level, the following section is presented for those who are interested in molecular genetic mechanisms.

The designation of "*1" for all of the cytochrome P450 genes is conventionally reserved for the "normal" form of a gene. Geneticists traditionally refer to this normal form of the gene as the *wild type* and consider all of the other variations as *mutants*. In the case of CYP2C19, the *1 allele produces an active form of the enzyme that is the "standard" by which the activity of the other CYP2C19 alleles is calibrated. Despite this convention, there are three versions of the *1 allele (e.g., *1A, *1B, and *1C). The *1C allele varies from the *1A allele as a result of an adenine to guanine change at nucleotide location 80161 in exon 7 (see Table 5.2). The *1B allele varies from the *1C allele by a cytosine to thymine change at nucleotide location 99 in exon 1, which means that it varies from *1A by two single nucleotide polymorphisms (SNPs). All three of these alleles produce an active form of the 2C19 enzyme.

The *2 allele varies from the *1B allele by a guanine to adenine change at nucleotide location 19154 in exon 5. Because this mutation results in a splicing defect that leads to termination of the synthesis of the enzyme, the protein produced by the *2 allele has no enzymatic activity. There is also a second change from the *1B allele, which is a cytosine to thymine change at nucleotide location 80160 in exon 7.

(*Continued*)

The *3 allele varies from the *1C allele by a guanine to adenine change at nucleotide location 17948 in exon 4. This results in the creation of a stop codon that leads to the formation of a truncated protein that has no enzymatic activity. There is also a second change from the *1C allele, which is an adenine to cytosine change at nucleotide location 87313 in exon 8.

The *4 allele has only one SNP variation from the *1B allele, which is an adenine to guanine change at nucleotide location 1 in the first exon. Since this mutation occurs in the initiation codon, it results in the inhibition of translation. Consequently, no active enzyme can be formed.

The *5 allele has only one SNP variation from the *1A allele, which is a cytosine to thymine change at nucleotide location 90033 in exon 9. This results in the creation of an unstable protein that has no enzymatic activity.

The *6 allele is differentiated from the *1B allele by a guanine to adenine change at nucleotide location 12748 in exon 3. This results in the creation of an unstable protein that has no enzymatic activity.

The *7 allele is identical to the *1A allele except for a thymine to adenine change at nucleotide location 19294 in intron 5 which results in an intron 5' splicing defect and the creation of a protein with no enzymatic activity.

The *8 allele is identical to the *1A allele except for a thymine to cytosine change at nucleotide location 12711 in exon 3. This results in the creation of an unstable protein that has no enzymatic activity.

The *9 allele is identical to the *1B allele with the exception of a guanine to adenine change at nucleotide location 12784 in exon 3. This results in the enzyme product having reduced activity.

The *10 allele is also identical to the *1B allele with the exception of a cytosine to thymine change at nucleotide location 19153 in exon 5. This results in the enzyme product having reduced activity.

The *17 allele is identical to the *1B allele with the exception of three variations in the promoter region of the gene at nucleotide locations −3402, −1041, and −806. These promoter changes result in the upregulation of gene expression. The *17 allele was first described in 2006 (Sim et al., 2006).

GENOTYPIC VARIANCE ACROSS GEOGRAPHIC ANCESTRY

The population frequency of CYP2C19 alleles varies dramatically across racial and ethnic groups. The pattern of this CYP2C19 variability provides insights into the process of human evolution. It also highlights the clinical utility of using genotyping to guide pharmacological decisions in patient populations of different geographic ancestry. Four population groups that have been more extensively studied will be described and contrasted to highlight the substantial variation of CYP2C19. The four populations reviewed are: 1) Northern Europeans, 2) Ethiopians, 3) Sub-Saharan

TABLE 5.2. CYP2C19 variations that define the 13 most common alleles

CYP2C19		5'FR			Exon 1		Exon 3			Exon 4	Exon 5		Intron 5	Exon 7		Exon 8	Exon 9
Allele	Enzyme Activity	−3402	−1041	−806	1	99	12711	12748	12784	17948	19153	19154	19294	80160	80161	87313	90033
*1A	Normal	C	A	C	A	C	T	G	G	G	C	G	T	C	A	A	C
*1B	Normal	C	A	C	A	T	T	G	G	G	C	G	T	C	G	A	C
*1C	Normal	C	A	C	A	C	T	G	G	G	C	G	T	C	G	A	C
*2	None	C	A	C	A	T	T	G	G	G	C	A	T	T	G	A	C
*3	None	C	A	C	A	C	T	G	G	A	C	G	T	C	G	C	C
*4	None	C	A	C	G	T	T	G	G	G	C	G	T	C	G	A	C
*5	None	C	A	C	A	C	T	G	G	G	C	G	T	C	A	A	C
*6	None	C	A	C	A	T	T	A	G	G	C	G	T	C	G	A	T
*7	None	C	A	C	A	C	T	G	G	G	C	G	A	C	A	A	C
*8	None	C	A	C	A	C	C	G	G	G	C	G	T	C	A	A	C
*9	Decreased	C	A	C	A	T	T	G	A	G	C	G	T	C	G	A	C
*10	Decreased	C	A	C	A	T	T	G	G	G	T	G	T	C	G	A	C
*17	Increased	T	G	T	A	T	T	G	G	G	C	G	T	C	G	A	C

This table documents the specific nucleotide variations that define common alleles of CYP2C19. Each row represents an allele, which is designated by a "*" and a number only. Each column represents a location on the gene map. The *1A row is the "wild type" reference sequence. The *1B and *1C alleles are variations of the *1A wild type allele that code for a completely functional form of the CYP2C19 enzyme. The nucleotides that are shaded represent variations from the "wild type" reference sequence.

TABLE 5.3. Variability in key allele frequencies in four groups with different geographical ancestry

Geographic Ancestry	*1 (%)	*2 (%)	*3 (%)	*17 (%)
Northern European	67	14	<1	18
Ethiopian	67	12	3	18
Sub-Saharan African	80	16	4	Unknown
Chinese	59	31	6	4

Africans, and 4) Chinese (Table 5.3). The allelic variation across these four geographic populations illustrates the challenges of using self-report of ethnicity or race to guide treatment. The precise allele frequencies for these specific alleles can be quite different in small communities within these large geographic regions because of variable migration, admixture, and persistent isolation (Dadds et al., 1999; Ingelman-Sundberg, 2005).

Northern Europeans

Northern European patients have a much lower frequency of inactive alleles than the Chinese. Specifically, only about 2% of European patients are poor CYP2C19 metabolizers, and about 26% are intermediate metabolizers (Xie et al., 1999). Consequently, psychiatrists treating patients in Northern Europe will develop a clinical impression that most of their patients will require the usual recommended dosage of amitriptyline or diazepam. However, a quarter of their patients will require a reduced dose, and about 2% of their patients will be unlikely to tolerate either of these two medications at recommended doses. The allele frequency of a newly identified *17 allele has been determined to be 18% in a Swedish population.

Ethiopians

Ethiopian patients have similar allele frequencies of CYP2C19*1 and CYP2C19*2 as Northern Europeans. However, the CYP2C19*3 allele is somewhat more common. The allele frequency of the newly identified CYP2C19*17 allele in Ethiopians is 18%, which is the same frequency found in Northern European samples.

Sub-Saharan Africans

Sub-Saharan Africans have not been studied as extensively, and the allele frequency of the newly reported CYP2C19*17 allele is unknown. However, there is a modest increase in the frequency of inactive alleles when compared to Northern Europeans.

Chinese

Chinese patients have a relatively high frequency of inactive CYP2C19 alleles. Specifically, about 25% of Chinese patients are poor metabolizers, while about another 50% are intermediate metabolizers. If patients have two inactive copies of CYP2C19, they will produce no normal 2C19 enzyme.

Psychiatrists treating patients in China learn that most of their patients will require quite modest doses of amitriptyline or diazepam, and that many of their patients will not be able to tolerate these two medications at any conventional dose. Only one in four Chinese patients will require a dose that is equivalent to that given the "average" European patient.

DEFINING CYP2C19 Metabolic Phenotypes

Individuals have only two copies of CYP2C19 as duplications of multiple copies of CYP2C19 on chromosome 10 have not been described. Traditionally, the full range of possible CYP2C19 genotypes has been classified into only three clinical CYP2C19 phenotypes. These were the poor metabolizer phenotype, the intermediate metabolizer phenotype, and the extensive metabolizer phenotype. However, with the discovery of the *17 allele, it is now possible to identify a new ultra-rapid metabolizer phenotype (Sim et al., 2006).

As in the case of CYP2D6, considerable confusion has been generated in the literature because different methodologies have been used to determine phenotypic classification based on genotypic differences. Once again, for the sake of clarity, the two common methods will be referred to as the current method and the historical method. The current methodology classifies more patients as intermediate metabolizers. For example, 1% of the Sequenced Treatment Alternatives to Relieve Depression (Star*D) study sample who have been classified as extensive metabolizers using the historical method would be reclassified as intermediate metabolizers using the current method. Using the current method, more patients are considered to be at risk for side effects of 2C19 substrate medication and would be more carefully monitored when taking these medications.

Again, the current method will henceforth be used, as it has become the standard. This is also the method widely used to describe dosage modifications of the psychotropic medications based on genotype (Kirchheiner et al., 2004).

The current definition of the poor metabolizer phenotype is an individual who has two inactive copies of CYP2C19, whereas the current definition of an intermediate metabolizer is an individual with one active copy and one inactive copy of CYP2C19. Extensive CYP2C19 metabolizers are individuals with two fully active copies of CYP2C19, or one active allele and one copy of the *17 allele. The three fully active CYP2C19 alleles are the *1 alleles (i.e., *1A, *1B, and *1C). The current definition of an ultra-rapid CYP2C19 metabolizer is an individual with two *17 alleles. Ultra-rapid CYP2C19 metabolizers have only quite recently been identified, and relatively little information is known about how these individuals metabolize most 2C19 substrate medications. However, the amount of 2C19 enzyme produced by the *17 allele is greater than the *1 alleles. This could explain the variability in response in patients who have historically been classified as *1/*1 extensive metabolizers of 2C19 substrate medications (Sim et al., 2006). Further research is needed to better characterize the phenotype metabolic function of both *1/*17 heterozygotes and *17/*17 homozygotes.

Antidepressant Medications

A number of antidepressants are metabolized primarily or partially by the 2C19 enzyme (Table 5.4). Specifically, amitriptyline, citalopram, clomipramine, and escitalopram are metabolized primarily by 2C19 (Herrlin et al., 2003; Kirchheiner et al., 2004; Steimer et al., 2004; Ulrich et al., 2001). In contrast, doxepin, imipramine, moclobemide, nortriptyline, and sertraline have substantial, but not exclusive, 2C19 substrate metabolic clearance. Venlafaxine is minimally metabolized by the 2C19 enzyme.

Antipsychotic Medications

The 2C19 enzyme plays a relatively circumscribed role in the metabolism of antipsychotic medications. It is substantially involved in the metabolism of clozapine and plays a minimal role in the metabolism of thioridazine.

TABLE 5.4. Antidepressant medications metabolized by the 2C19 enzyme

Antidepressant Medications Primarily Metabolized by 2C19	Antidepressant Medications Substantially Metabolized by 2C19	Antidepressant Medications Minimally Metabolized by 2C19
Amitriptyline	Doxepin	Venlafaxine
Citalopram	Imipramine	
Clomipramine	Moclobemide	
Escitalopram	Nortriptyline	
	Sertraline	

ANXIOLYTIC MEDICATIONS

The 2C19 enzyme plays a primary role in the metabolism of diazepam. The role of this enzyme in the metabolism of other benzodiazepines has not been well demonstrated.

PROTEIN-PUMP INHIBITORS

The 2C19 enzyme plays a primary role in the metabolism of most protein-pump inhibitors that have been used to treat patients with increased gastric acid secretion. These include lansoprazole, omeprazole, and pantoprazole.

CLINICAL IMPLICATIONS

The current clinical applications of CYP2C19 genotyping are similar to those discussed for CYP2D6 genotyping in Chapter 4. Poor metabolizers can be given either an alternative medication that is not a 2C19 substrate medication or their dose can be started at a low level and titrated slowly. If these patients can tolerate a standard dose, their serum level will be higher than that of a patient who has an extensive metabolizer phenotype, and this elevated serum level may be associated with a good therapeutic response. Patients with an intermediate metabolizer phenotype may tolerate the standard doses of 2C19 substrate medications or may require a modest decrease in dose. Patients with the extensive or normal metabolizer phenotype may be prescribed 2C19 substrate medications as directed. Finally, patients with the ultra-rapid CYP2C19 metabolizer phenotype will require higher doses of 2C19 substrate medications to achieve therapeutic serum levels. These patients should be closely monitored if higher doses are prescribed.

The clinical utility of CYP2C19 genotyping must be assessed according to the degree of genetic variability that exists within a given clinical population. The clinical utility of the CYP2C19 genotyping for identifying poor metabolizers is much greater in Chinese populations than in Northern European populations because of the frequency of inactive alleles. If we consider a single drug, such as amitriptyline, in Chinese patients about 50% will have a direct benefit for pharmacogenomic testing. This estimate is based on the expectation that psychiatrists treating primarily Chinese patients will need to modify their dosing strategy so that it will be beneficial for the "average" Chinese patient. In China, the "average" patient is actually an intermediate 2C19 metabolizer. If genotyping was not available, it would make good clinical sense to provide all Chinese patients with an initial low dose. Unfortunately, this strategy would result in about 25% of Chinese patients having an increased risk for side effects, even when their initial dose of amitriptyline is relatively low. However, the Chinese patients who are the most disadvantaged by this dosing strategy are those who are currently classified as having extensive metabolism based on the fact that they have two normal copies of CYP2C19. Such patients are unlikely to respond to the lower doses of amitriptyline that would be well tolerated by intermediate CYP2C19 metabolizers. Of course, competent clinicians can ultimately titrate the dose of amitriptyline up to a level that is effective for their patients who are extensive metabolizers. If extensive metabolizers who do not respond to the initial treatment are able to tolerate the gradual titration of their dose upward, they will eventually reach an adequate serum level, and their depression may improve. However, unless their amitriptyline serum level is monitored, a risk exists that either the patient or his psychiatrist will become impatient with the absence of a therapeutic response and abandon treatment with amitriptyline before an adequate serum level is achieved. By monitoring the amitriptyline serum levels of these patients, the appropriate dose, as well as the adherence of the patient, can be determined. In summary, a single determination of the CYP2C19 genotype can allow a reasonably accurate prediction of the phenotype of the patient. Ongoing monitoring of tricyclic antidepressant serum levels can provide patient-specific documentation for the most appropriate dose of medication.

Clinical Implications of CYP2C19*17

The degree of clinical benefit that can be achieved by using CYP2C19 genotyping to identify patients who will not respond to usual doses of 2C19 substrate medication in a community is dependent on the frequency of genetic variations that increase the functional capacity of CYP2C19 within the population. Until the discovery of the CYP2C19*17 allele, it was not possible to identify ultra-rapid 2C19 metabolizers. However, it is now known that the allele frequency of the CYP2C19*17 allele is 18% in Northern Europeans and 4% in Chinese. Consequently, about 4% of Northern Europeans are ultra-rapid 2C19 metabolizers, whereas 9% have a somewhat accelerated 2C19 metabolism. Only 0.2% of Chinese patients are ultra-rapid 2C19 metabolizers, whereas about 1% has an accelerated 2C19 metabolism. Since the frequency of ultra-rapid 2C19 metabolizers among Northern Europeans is considerably higher than that in the Chinese, adding the CYP2C19*17 allele to pharmacogenomic genotyping will improve the clinical utility of the test more when treating Northern European patients than Chinese patients.

Clinical Case 2

A 40-year-old professional woman had been treated for her depression and anxiety since she was 18. Over these 22 years, she had been prescribed 11 antidepressants by four different psychiatrists. During this time, she had experienced a wide range of unpleasant side effects, but she had been repeatedly encouraged to keep taking her medications. Her medical record included many comments suggesting that she was probably noncompliant and that she had exaggerated the severity of her side effects. The patient noted that her sister was also sensitive to antidepressants and that her sister had essentially given up any hope of finding an effective treatment. Her psychiatrist ordered pharmacogenomic testing (Table 5.5).

TABLE 5.5. Pharmacogenomic report of case 2

Pharmacogenomic Report of Case 2		
Gene	Genotype	Clinical Implication
CYP2D6	*5/*5	Poor CYP2D6 metabolizer
CYP2C19	*2/*2	Poor CYP2C19 metabolizer

Genotyping revealed that the patient was a poor metabolizer of both CYP2D6 and CYP2C19. Ironically, the patient had never been treated with fluvoxamine, which is not primarily metabolized by either the 2D6 or the 2C19 enzyme. The patient was prescribed fluvoxamine, which she was able to tolerate, and her symptoms of depression substantially resolved. The patient subsequently took considerable pleasure in explaining to her previous psychiatrists that her quite rare genotype made it virtually impossible for her to tolerate the medications that they had prescribed for her.

Her sister was subsequently genotyped and was also determined to be a poor metabolizer of both CYP2D6 and CYP2C19. She similarly had a good response to treatment with fluvoxamine.

Clinical Case 3

A 32-year-old Chinese woman developed severe depressive symptoms. Her symptoms included an inability to fall asleep and daily early morning awakening. She was placed on 25 mg of amitriptyline in the morning and evening. After her first evening dose, she slept well for the first time in several weeks. However, her mouth was quite dry when she awoke. By the third day of treatment, she had developed a severe headache and felt quite sedated. Her psychiatrist ordered CYP2D6 and CYP2C19 genotypes (Table 5.6) and an amitriptyline serum level. Her combined serum level of amitriptyline and its metabolite, nortriptyline, was found to be 300 ng/mL. This was above the recommended range of the laboratory (Ulrich et al., 2001). Her psychiatrist subsequently decreased her dose to 10 mg.

(*Continued*)

TABLE 5.6. Pharmacogenomic report of case 3

Pharmacogenomic Report of Case 3		
Gene	Genotype	Clinical Implication
CYP2D6	*1/*2A	Extensive CYP2D6 metabolizer
CYP2C19	*3/*3	Poor CYP2C19 metabolizer

The following day, her pharmacogenomic report revealed that the CYP2C19 genotype of the patient was *3/*3, but that she was an extensive metabolizer of 2D6 substrate medication with a *1/*2A genotype. Her psychiatrist subsequently prescribed a low dose of nortriptyline, which is primarily metabolized by the 2D6 enzyme. However, he chose to monitor her serum levels to establish the appropriate dose given that she was a poor CYP2C19 metabolizer and the 2C19 enzyme can play a secondary role in the metabolism of nortriptyline.

Clinical Case 4

A 45-year-old Swedish woman presented to her psychiatrist with intermittent periods of intense anxiety. She described episodes of generalized anxiety that would last for 2 to 3 days and then resolve. She reportedly experienced one of these prolonged periods of anxiety about once every month. This patient had been treated with citalopram and fluvoxamine without receiving significant benefit. After several years of not receiving effective treatment for her anxiety, she discovered that if she took diazepam at the time of the onset of her anxiety, her symptoms would resolve reasonably quickly. However, she required a dose of at least 40 mg of diazepam a day to achieve this relief from her symptoms. Her psychiatrist was concerned that she would become dependent on diazepam if she insisted on taking this high dose. He subsequently ordered pharmacogenomic testing to clarify her CYP2C19 and CYP2D6 genotype (Table 5.7).

TABLE 5.7. Pharmacogenomic report of case 4

Pharmacogenomic Report of Case 4		
Gene	Genotype	Clinical Implication
CYP2D6	*1/*1	Extensive CYP2D6 metabolizer
CYP2C19	*17/*17	Ultra-Rapid CYP2C19 metabolizer

Pharmacogenomic testing revealed that this patient had a CYP2C19 genotype of *17/*17 and was an ultra-rapid 2C19 metabolizer. Testing also documented that she was an extensive CYP2D6 metabolizer. Her CYP2C19 genotype provided a rational explanation for her capacity to benefit from high doses of diazepam without experiencing the level of side effects that would be anticipated to occur when taking these high doses.

KEY CLINICAL CONSIDERATIONS

For patients with the CYP2C19 *poor metabolizer phenotype*:

- Avoid using 2C19 substrate medications or use these medications at lower than the recommended doses and monitor the patient closely for side effects.

For patients with the CYP2C19 *intermediate metabolizer phenotype*:

- Use 2C19 substrate medications at lower than recommended doses.

For patients with the CYP2C19 *ultra-rapid metabolizer phenotype*:

- Avoid using 2C19 substrate medications or use these medications at increased doses, while carefully monitoring the patient in order to be able to recognize adverse reactions that may result from high serum levels of secondary metabolites.

REFERENCES

Dadds, M. R., Holland, D. E., Laurens, K. R., Mullins, M., Barrett, P. M., & Spence, S. H. (1999). Early intervention and prevention of anxiety disorders in children: results at 2-year follow-up. *Journal of Consulting & Clinical Psychology, 67*(1), 145–150.

Goldstein, J. A., & de Morais, S. M. (1994). Biochemistry and molecular biology of the human CYP2C subfamily. *Pharmacogenetics, 4*(6), 285–299.

Herrlin, K., Yasui-Furukori, N., Tybring, G., Widen, J., Gustafsson, L. L., & Bertilsson, L. (2003). Metabolism of citalopram enantiomers in CYP2C19/CYP2D6 phenotyped panels of healthy Swedes. *British Journal of Clinical Pharmacology, 56*(4), 415–421.

Ingelman-Sundberg, M. (2005). Genetic polymorphisms of cytochrome P450 2D6 (CYP2D6): clinical consequences, evolutionary aspects, and functional diversity. *Pharmacogenomics Journal, 5*(1), 6–13.

Kirchheiner, J., Heesch, C., Bauer, S., Meisel, C., Seringer, A., Goldammer, M., et al. (2004). Impact of the ultrarapid metabolizer genotype of cytochrome P450 2D6 on metoprolol pharmacokinetics and pharmacodynamics. *Clinical Pharmacology and Therapeutics, 76*, 302–312.

Kirchheiner, J., Nickchen, K., Bauer, M., Wong, M.-L., Licinio, J., Roots, I., & Brockmoller, J. (2004). Pharmacogenetics of antidepressants and antipsychotics: the contribution of allelic variations to the phenotype of drug response. *Molecular Psychiatry, 9*, 442–473.

Kupfer, A., Desmond, P., Schenker, S., & Branch, R. (1979). Family study of a genetically determined deficiency of mephenytoin hydroxylation in man. [letter]. *Pharmacologist, 21*(173).

Sim, S. C., Risinger, C., Dahl, M. L., Aklillu, E., Christensen, M., Bertilsson, L., & Ingelman-Sundberg, M. (2006). A common novel CYP2C19 gene variant causes ultrarapid drug metabolism relevant for the drug response to proton pump inhibitors and antidepressants. *Clinical Pharmacology and Therapeutics, 79*(1), 103–113.

Steimer, W., Zopf, K., Von Amelunxen, S., Pfeiffer, H., Bachofer, J., Popp, J., et al. (2004). Allele-specific change of concentration and functional gene dose for the prediction of steady-state serum concentrations of amitriptyline and nortriptyline in CYP2C19 and CY2D6 extensive and intermediate metabolizers. *Clinical Chemistry, 50*(9), 1623–1633.

Ulrich, S., Northoff, G., Wurthmann, C., Partscht, G., Pester, U., Herscu, H., & Meyer, F. P. (2001). Serum levels of amitriptyline and therapeutic effect in non-delusional moderately to severely depressed in-patients: a therapeutic window relationship. *Pharmacopsychiatry, 34*(1), 33–40.

Wrighton, S. A., Stevens, J. C., Becker, G. W., & VandenBranden, M. (1993). Isolation and characterization of human liver cytochrome P450 2C19: correlation between 2C19 and S-mephenytoin 4'-hydroxylation. *Archives of Biochemistry & Biophysics, 306*(1), 240–245.

Xie, H. G., Stein, C. M., Kim, R. B., Wilkinson, G. R., Flockhart, D. A., & Wood, A. J. (1999). Allelic, genotypic and phenotypic distributions of S-mephenytoin 4'-hydroxylase (CYP2C19) in healthy Caucasian populations of European descent throughout the world. *Pharmacogenetics, 9*(5), 539–549.

WEBSITES

Karolinska Institute: Human Cytochrome P450 (*CYP*) Allele Nomenclature Committee   http://www.cypalleles.ki.se/

6

THE CYTOCHROME P450 2C9 GENE

The cytochrome P450 2C9 gene (CYP2C9) codes for an enzyme that facilitates the oxidation of about 100 medications. These include drugs with a narrow therapeutic index, such as warfarin and phenytoin, as well as many of the nonsteroidal antiinflammatory drugs (NSAIDs). Amitriptyline and fluoxetine are substantially metabolized by CYP2C9 and the 2C9 enzyme can play an important role in drug clearance, if the primary metabolic pathway is nonfunctional.

LOCATION AND GENE VARIATION

CYP2C9 is located on chromosome 10 just proximal to CYP2C19. The specific location of the gene is on the long arm of chromosome 10 at 10q24 (Fig. 6.1).

CYP2C9 consists of approximately 50,708 nucleotides or 50.7 kilobases. It contains nine exons, as does CYP2C19. The exons in CYP2C9 are composed of 1,835 nucleotides, and the gene codes for a polypeptide that is composed of 490 amino acids (Fig. 6.2).

Table 6.1 provides a list of the commonly identified CYP2C9 alleles, their activity levels, and their estimated allele frequency in Northern European populations.

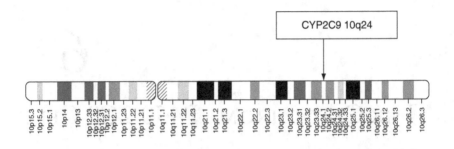

FIGURE 6.1. Chromosome 10 with arrow to designate the location of CYP2C9.

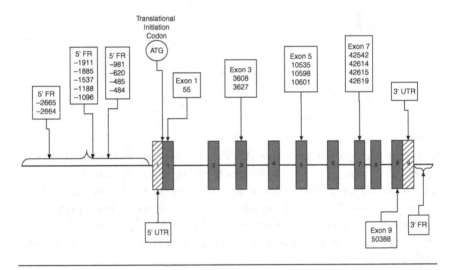

FIGURE 6.2. CYP2C9 structure illustrating the location of the nine exons and the single nucleotide polymorphisms that define the most important 2C9 alleles.

Technical Discussion of CYP2C9 Variations (see Fig. 6.2 and Tables 6.1 and 6.2)

Each of the most well-studied CYP2C9 alleles is described in this technical discussion. Although clinicians do not need to learn the precise nucleotide changes that influence CYP2C9 enzyme activity level, the following section is presented for those who are interested in molecular genetic mechanisms.

CYP2C9 is a highly variable gene. Currently there are 37 known variants, although only 12 distinct alleles have been given a * designation. Table 6.1 lists the 12 relatively common CYP2C9 variations that can be identified by clinical reference laboratories, although some clinical laboratories only genotype *1, *2, and

*3. Table 6.1 also includes the activity level of the gene products that each of these alleles produce. Table 6.2 shows the specific variations of the genes and the location of variable single nucleotide polymorphisms (SNPs).

The CYP2C9*1A allele is the normal or wild type allele of CYP2C9.

The CYP2C9*2A, CYP2C9*2B, and CYP2C9*2C alleles all produce a protein product that has a decreased enzyme activity (Shintani et al., 2001).

The CYP2C9*2A allele has five SNPs in the 5' region (i.e., –1188 thymine to cytosine, –1096 adenine to guanine, –620 guanine to thymine, –485 thymine to adenine, and –484 cytosine to adenine) and a 3608 cytosine to thymine change in exon 3.

The CYP2C9*2B allele and the CYP2C9*11B allele have a deletion of thymine at the –2665 nucleotide location and a deletion of guanine at the –2664 nucleotide location in the 5' region. The five SNPs located in the 5' region and the 3608 cytosine to thymine change in exon 3 are common to all three of the CYP2C9*2 alleles.

The CYP2C9*2C allele shares the common variants of the CYP2C9*2A alleles with the exception of the thymine to cytosine change at the –1188 nucleotide location in the 5' region.

The two most common forms of CYP2C9*3 are designated as CYP2C9*3A and CYP2C9*3B, and both of these alleles produce a form of the CYP2C9 enzyme with decreased activity. Both have a set of four SNPs (i.e., –1911 thymine to cytosine, –1885 cytosine to guanine, –1537 guanine to adenine, and –981 guanine to adenine at the 5'-flanking region, as well as a common adenine to cytosine SNP at the 42614 nucleotide location in exon 7. Additionally, CYP2C9*3B also has a thymine to cytosine change at nucleotide location –1188 in the 5' region.

The CYP2C9*4 allele is the result of a thymine to cytosine change at nucleotide location 42615 in exon 7, and the activity level of the gene product is not known.

The CYP2C9*5 allele is the result of a cytosine to guanine change at nucleotide location 42619 in exon 7 and produces a form of the CYP2C9 enzyme with reduced activity.

The genetic variants that define CYP2C9*3, CYP2C9*4, and CYP2C9*5 allelic variants are all located within exon 7 and are believed to reside within the putative substrate recognition site 5 of the CYP2 family. This is an important region for substrate binding (Xie et al., 2002).

The CYP2C9*6 allele is the result of a rare single adenine deletion near the 3' end of exon 5 at nucleotide location 10601 and produces a form of the CYP2C9 enzyme with no activity.

The CYP2C9*7 allele is the result of a cytosine to adenine change at nucleotide location 55 in exon 1 and has an undetermined effect on enzyme activity level.

The CYP2C9*8 allele is the result of a guanine to adenine change at nucleotide location 3627 in exon 3. The CYP2C9*8 allele produces a form of the CYP2C9 enzyme with somewhat increased activity.

The CYP2C9*9 allele is the result of an adenine to guanine change at nucleotide location 10535 in exon 5. The CYP2C9*9 allele produces a form of the CYP2C9 enzyme with slightly decreased enzyme activity.

The CYP2C9*10 allele is the result of an adenine to guanine change at nucleotide location 10598 in exon 5. The CYP2C9*10 allele produces a form of the CYP2C9 enzyme with slightly decreased enzyme activity.

(*Continued*)

The CYP2C9*11A allele is the result of a cytosine to thymine change at nucleotide location 42542 in exon 7. This results in a folding problem in the structure of the CYP2C9 protein that results in the production of a CYP2C9 enzyme with decreased activity.

The CYP2C9*11B allele has a deletion of a thymine at the −2665 nucleotide location and a deletion of a guanine at the −2664 nucleotide location in the 5' region. These two deletions also occur in the CYP2C9*2B allele. The CYP2C9*11B allele also has a thymine to cytosine change at nucleotide location −1188 in the 5' region and a cytosine to thymine change at nucleotide location 42542 in exon 7. This nucleotide change at nucleotide location 42542 in exon 7 also occurs in the CYP2C9*11A allele. The CYP2C9*11B allele produces a form of the CYP2C9 enzyme with decreased activity.

The CYP2C9*12 allele is the result of a cytosine to thymine change at nucleotide location 50388 in exon 9. This results in the production of a form of the CYP2C9 enzyme with decreased activity (Blaisdell et al., 2004).

TABLE 6.1. The activity level of the 12 commonly genotyped 2C9 alleles and their European allele frequency

Allele	Activity Level	Northern European Allele Frequency(%)
*1A	Normal	74–86
*2A, *2B, *2C	Decreased	8–19
*3A, *3B	Decreased	3–16
*4	Unknown	<1
*5	Decreased	<0.1
*6	None	<1
*7	Unknown	<1
*8	Increased	<1
*9	Decreased	<1
*10	Decreased	<1
*11A, *11B	Decreased	1
*12	Decreased	<1

Xie et al. (2001); Mizutani, T. (2003) and Suarez-Kurtz (2005).

GENOTYPIC VARIANCE ACROSS GEOGRAPHIC ANCESTRY

The CYP2C9*1 allele is the most common allele in most geographic ancestral groups (Table 6.3).

TABLE 6.2. CYP2C9 variations that define 16 common alleles

CYP2C9	5' FR											Exon 1	Exon 3		Exon 5				Exon 7			Exon 9
Allele	-2665	-2664	-1911	-1885	-1537	-1188	-1096	-981	-620	-485	-484	55	3608	3627	10535	10598	10601	42542	42614	42615	42619	50388
*1A	T	G	T	C	G	T	A	G	G	T	C	C	C	G	A	A	A	C	A	T	C	C
*2A	T	G	T	C	G	C	G	G	T	A	A	C	T	G	A	A	A	C	A	T	C	C
*2B	Deletion of TG		T	C	G	C	G	G	T	A	A	C	T	G	A	A	A	C	A	T	C	C
*2C	T	G	T	C	G	T	G	G	T	A	A	C	T	G	A	A	A	C	A	T	C	C
*3A	T	G	C	G	A	A	A	A	G	T	C	C	C	G	A	A	A	C	C	T	C	C
*3B	T	G	C	G	A	C	A	A	G	T	C	C	C	G	A	A	A	C	C	T	C	C
*4	T	G	T	C	G	T	A	G	G	T	C	C	C	G	A	A	A	C	A	C	C	C
*5	T	G	T	C	G	T	A	G	G	T	C	C	C	G	A	A	A	C	A	T	G	C
*6	T	G	T	C	G	T	A	G	G	T	C	A	C	G	A	A	Delete A	C	A	T	C	C
*7	T	G	T	C	G	T	A	G	G	T	C	C	C	A	A	A	A	C	A	T	C	C
*8	T	G	T	C	G	T	A	G	G	T	C	C	C	G	G	A	A	C	A	T	C	C
*9	T	G	T	C	G	T	A	G	G	T	C	C	C	G	A	G	A	C	A	T	C	C
*10	T	G	T	C	G	T	A	G	G	T	C	C	C	G	A	G	A	C	A	T	C	C
*11A	T	G	T	C	G	T	A	G	G	T	C	C	C	G	A	A	A	T	A	T	C	C
*11B	Deletion of TG		T	C	G	C	A	G	G	T	C	C	C	G	A	A	A	T	A	T	C	C
*12	T	G	T	C	G	T	A	G	G	T	C	C	C	G	A	A	A	C	A	T	C	T

This table documents the specific nucleotide variations that define the common alleles of CYP2C9. Each row represents an allele, which is designated by a "*" with a number and letter, or a "*" with a number only. Each column represents a location on the gene map. The *1A row is the "wild-type" reference sequence. Shaded nucleotides represent variations from the wild-type reference sequence.

TABLE 6.3. Variability in allele frequencies in four geographical populations

Geographic Ancestry	*1 (%)	*2 (%)	*3 (%)	*5 (%)
Northern European	74–86	8–19	3–16	<0.1
Sub-Saharan African	95	<0.1	<0.1	1–2
Ethiopian	93	4	2	<0.1
Chinese	95–98	<0.1	1–5	<0.1

These allele frequencies are based on multiple reports in the literature. Suarez-Kurtz (2005).

Northern Europeans

Considerable variability in the CYP2C9*2 allele frequency exists among many European populations with a range of CYP2C9*2 allele frequency from 8% to 19%. Europeans also have considerable variation in the allele frequency of CYP2C9*3 with a range of 3% to 16%.

Ethiopians

The CYP2C9*2 allele frequency of 4% and the CYP2C9*3 allele frequency of 2% is less common in Ethiopians than in Europeans (Seng et al., 2003).

Sub-Saharan Africans

The CYP2C9*5 allele has been identified in Sub-Saharan Tanzanians and Beninese, but it has not been identified in Europeans, Ethiopians, or Chinese populations (Suarez-Kurtz, 2005).

Chinese

In Chinese populations, the allele frequencies of the CYP2C9*3 allele ranges between 1% and 5%. The CYP2C9*2, CYP2C9*4, and CYP2C9*5 alleles are rarer in Chinese populations (Si et al., 2004).

DEFINING 2C9 METABOLIC PHENOTYPES

About 8–11% of subjects of European ancestry are poor metabolizers of CYP2C9 substrates. This phenotype is defined by having either two alleles with deficient activity, one allele with deficient activity and one allele with no activity, or two alleles with no activity (Xie et al., 2001). Given that the frequency of CYP2C9 alleles that produce CYP2C9 enzyme with no activity is <1% in Caucasians and even rarer in Asians, most poor metabolizers can produce some functional enzyme. However, the clinical consequence of having two CYP2C9 alleles with no activity can be quite serious and includes life-threatening bleeding episodes following administration of warfarin and severe toxicity with phenytoin administration (Danielson, 2002).

ANTIDEPRESSANT MEDICATIONS

Amitriptyline

Amitriptyline is a tricyclic antidepressant that is demethylated by both CYP2C9 and CYP3A4 to produce nortriptyline, which is an active metabolite (Ghahramani et al., 1997). Amitriptyline is hydroxylated by CYP2D6 (Kirchheiner et al., 2003).

Fluoxetine

Fluoxetine is a selective serotonin reuptake inhibitor (SSRI) that is metabolized primarily via N-demethylation by CYP2D6. Demethylation results in the production of norfluoxetine, which is also biologically active. Fluoxetine is metabolized secondarily by CYP2C9. Given the slow elimination of fluoxetine and the subsequent required secondary clearance of norfluoxetine, fluoxetine has the longest functional half-life of any SSRI antidepressant.

Sertraline

Sertraline is an SSRI that is metabolized by five cytochrome P450 enzymes (i.e., CYP2D6, CYP2C9, CYP2B6, CYP2C19, and CYP3A4). Consequently, the inhibition of any single enzyme does not result in a major change in the pharmacokinetics of sertraline. However, poor CYP2C19 metabolizers have been shown to have higher serum levels of sertraline than do normal metabolizers at a standard dose. The inhibition of CYP2B6 is reported to have an equivalent effect. The contribution of CYP2C9 and CYP3A4 to sertraline metabolism is minimal unless there is impaired CYP2C19 and CYP2B6 metabolism capacity (Table 6.4). The major metabolite of sertraline, desmethylsertraline, is a weak serotonin transporter reuptake inhibitor.

TABLE 6.4. Antidepressant medications metabolized by the 2C9 enzyme

Antidepressants Primarily Metabolized by 2C9	Antidepressants Substantially Metabolized by 2C9	Antidepressants Minimally Metabolized by 2C9
None	Amitriptyline Fluoxetine	Sertraline

Other 2C9 Substrate Medications

Nonsteroidal Anti-Inflammatory Drugs (NSAIDs)

Celecoxib

Celecoxib is an NSAID that results in a decrease of prostaglandin synthesis. Celecoxib is a highly selective cyclooxygenase COX-2 inhibitor. Traditional NSAIDs inhibit both COX-1 and COX-2. Celecoxib is primarily metabolized by CYP2C9 enzyme (Fung & Kirschenbaum, 1999). The clearance of celecoxib is significantly reduced by CYP2C9*3, but not CYP2C9*2 (Perini et al., 2005).

Diclofenac

Diclofenac is an NSAID metabolized by CYP2C9. A hypothesized mechanism of action is the inhibition of prostaglandin synthesis by inhibition of both COX-1 and COX-2 (Rodrigues, 2005).

Ibuprofen

Ibuprofen is an NSAID metabolized by CYP2C9 (Rodrigues, 2005). Ibuprofen inhibits both COX-1 and COX-2, which results in a decrease of prostaglandin synthesis. The clearance of ibuprofen is significantly reduced by CYP2C9*3, but not CYP2C9*2 (Perini et al., 2005).

Lornoxicam

Lornoxicam is an NSAID primarily hydroxylated by CYP2C9. It also decreases prostaglandin synthesis by inhibiting COX and has a relatively short elimination half-life of 3–5 hours. The presence of a single inactive CYP2C9 allele has been shown to impair the oral clearance of lornoxicam (Zhang et al., 2005).

Naproxen

Naproxen is an NSAID that is oxidized by CYP2C9 and CYP1A2 (Rodrigues, 2005). This is in contrast to the oxidative metabolism of other NSAIDs, such as diclofenac and ibuprofen, which are almost exclusively metabolized by CYP2C9 (Miners et al., 1996).

Piroxicam

Piroxicam is an NSAID that is a nonselective COX inhibitor. CYP2C9 is the major pathway for the metabolism of piroxicam. Patients who are poor

CYP2C9 metabolizers have their clearance of piroxicam reduced up to 30-fold. In most cases, the effects of allele *3 on drug clearance were more marked than for those of allele *2.

Suprofen

Suprofen is an NSAID that, like ibuprofen and naproxen, is a 2-arylpropionic acid compound. Suprofen oxidation is primarily metabolized by CYP2C9 (Mancy, et al., 1995). Unlike other NSAIDs, suprofen has been known to cause adverse drug reactions related to acute renal failure. The acute flank pain syndrome associated with these reactions typically occurred within a few hours of administration of suprofen (O'Donnell et al., 2003).

Antidiabetic Medications

Glipizide

Glipizide is a second-generation sulfonylurea antidiabetic drug that undergoes enterohepatic circulation. The proposed mechanism of action of glipizide is to block potassium channels in the β-cells of the islets of Langerhans. The oral clearance of glipizide in a poor metabolizer of CYP2C9 was only 20% of the rate of patients who are CYP2C9 extensive metabolizers (Kirchheiner et al., 2005).

Glyburide

Glyburide is a sulfonylurea antidiabetic agent that stimulates insulin release. CYP2C9 plays a major role in the biotransformation of glyburide in humans, but not CYP2D6 or CYP2C19 (Kirchheiner et al., 2005).

Nateglinide

Nateglinide is a drug in the meglitinide class that lowers blood glucose by stimulating the release of insulin from the pancreas. Nateglinide is primarily metabolized by CYP2C9. However, CYP2D6 and CYP1A2 are also involved in nateglinide metabolism (Kirchheiner et al., 2005).

Rosiglitazone

Rosiglitazone is an antidiabetic drug in the thiazolidinedione class of drugs, which is metabolized by CYP2C9 and CYP2C8 via demethylation (Kirchheiner et al., 2005). Recent findings suggest that rosiglitazone is associated with a statistically significant risk of cardiovascular disease events.

Angiotensin II Receptor Antagonist Drugs

Irbesartan

Irbesartan is an angiotensin II receptor antagonist used for the treatment of hypertension. CYP2C9 plays a major part in the metabolism of irbesartan. Diastolic blood pressure response differed in relation to the CYP2C9 genotype in patients given irbesartan. The reduction in patients with genotype CYP2C9*1/*1 was 7.5% compared to those with genotype CYP2C9*1/*2, which was 14.4%. A similar trend was seen for systolic blood pressure (Hallberg et al., 2002).

Losartan

Losartan is an angiotensin II receptor antagonist used for the treatment of hypertension and diabetic nephropathy. CYP2C9 is the primary enzyme that facilitates the metabolism of losartan (Hallberg et al., 2002), although CYP3A4 can also become involved in the metabolism of losartan at high serum concentrations (Yasar et al., 2001).

Phenytoin

Phenytoin is an antiepileptic that is also used in the treatment of trigeminal neuralgia. Phenytoin is metabolized by both CYP2C9 and CYP2C19. CYP2C9 is the primary metabolic pathway and accounts for between 70% and 90% of the total clearance of phenytoin (Murphy & Wilbur, 2003).

S-warfarin

Warfarin is an anticoagulant that is effective in the prophylaxis of thrombosis and embolism. Warfarin treatment must be monitored through frequent blood testing to track the international normalized ratio (INR), which is used to define an effective dose that will not result in bleeding.

Warfarin is a synthetic derivative of coumarin, which occurs naturally in plants. Warfarin consists of a racemic mixture of two active isomers, each of which is cleared by different pathways. However, the S-warfarin isomer has five times the potency of the R-isomer with respect to vitamin K antagonism.

Two genes are known to influence warfarin metabolism. The vitamin K epoxide reductase complex 1 (VKORC1) gene explains 30% of the dose variation between patients. Two haplotypes explain 25% of variation, and are referred to as the low-dose haplotype group (A) and the high-dose haplotype group (B). Variation of CYP2C9 is believed to account for another 10% of variation in warfarin dosing (Veenstra et al., 2005).

CLINICAL IMPLICATIONS

Genotyping of CYP2C9 has not been widely utilized in the care of psychiatric patients. However, the documentation of CYP2C9 genotypes can be important in psychiatric patients who are poor metabolizers of CYP2D6, CYP2C19, or CYP1A2. The following case illustrates the clinical relevance.

Clinical Case 5

A 17-year-old boy developed a serious depression after being rejected by the seven universities to which he had applied. His family physician prescribed a standard 20 mg dose of fluoxetine at bedtime. After his first dose, he experienced a sense of panic. After his second dose, he was unable to attend school because of severe headaches. After he took a third and final dose, he had difficulty sleeping and experienced the onset of severe diarrhea. His doctor advised him to discontinue taking his medication and ordered pharmacogenetic testing (Table 6.5).

TABLE 6.5. Pharmacogenomic report of case 5

Pharmacogenomic Report of Case 5		
Gene	Genotype of Patient	Clinical Implication
CYP2D6	*4/*4	Poor CYP2D6 metabolizer
CYP2C19	*1/*1	Extensive CYP2C19 metabolizer
CYP2C9	*3/*6	Poor CYP2C9 metabolizer

This patient experienced severe side effects to fluoxetine that could not fully be explained by the fact that he had no CYP2D6 enzyme activity. His symptoms were more severe and he experienced a more rapid onset of symptoms than is reported in most poor 2D6 metabolizers who have been prescribed fluoxetine. The most straightforward explanation for the severity of symptoms is that he was also a poor metabolizer of 2C9 substrates. Given that he had adequate levels of CYP2C19 enzyme, he would probably tolerate alternative antidepressants that were CYP2C19 substrates, such as citalopram. Unfortunately, because fluoxetine has a very long half-life, his uncomfortable symptoms persisted for several days.

KEY CLINICAL CONSIDERATIONS

- CYP2C9 can play a clinically significant role in the metabolism of amitriptyline, fluoxetine, and sertraline, if their primary metabolic pathway is not functional.

- CYP2C9 plays an important role in the metabolism of phenytoin and warfarin.

REFERENCES

Blaisdell, J., Jorge-Nebert, L. F., Coulter, S., Ferguson, S. S., Lee, S. J., Chanas, B., et al. (2004). Discovery of new potentially defective alleles of human CYP2C9. *Pharmacogenetics, 14*(8), 527–537.

Danielson, P. B. (2002). The cytochrome P450 superfamily: biochemistry, evolution and drug metabolism in humans. *Current Drug Metabolism, 3*(6), 561–597.

Fung, H. B., & Kirschenbaum, H. L. (1999). Selective cyclooxygenase-2 inhibitors for the treatment of arthritis. *Clinical Therapeutics, 21*(7), 1131–1157.

Ghahramani, P., Ellis, S. W., Lennard, M. S., Ramsay, L. E., & Tucker, G. T. (1997). Cytochromes P450 mediating the N-demethylation of amitriptyline. *British Journal of Clinical Psychology, 43*(2), 137–144.

Hallberg, P., Karlsson, J., Kurland, L., Lind, L., Kahan, T., Malmqvist, K., et al. (2002). The CYP2C9 genotype predicts the blood pressure response to irbesartan: results from the Swedish Irbesartan Left Ventricular Hypertrophy Investigation vs Atenolol (SILVHIA) trial. *Journal of Hypertension, 20*(10), 2089–2093.

Kirchheiner, J., Muller, G., Meineke, I., Wernecke, K. D., Roots, I., & Brockmoller, J. (2003). Effects of polymorphisms in CYP2D6, CYP2C9, and CYP2C19 on trimipramine pharmacokinetics. *Journal of Clinical Psychopharmacology, 23*(5), 459–466.

Kirchheiner, J., Roots, I., Goldammer, M., Rosenkranz, B., & Brockmoller, J. (2005). Effect of genetic polymorphisms in cytochrome p450 (CYP) 2C9 and CYP2C8 on the pharmacokinetics of oral antidiabetic drugs: clinical relevance. *Clinical pharmacokinetics, 44*(12), 1209–1225.

Mancy, A., Broto, P., Dijols, S., Dansette, P. M., & Mansuy, D. (1995). The substrate binding site of human liver cytochrome P450 2C9: an approach using designed tienilic acid derivatives and molecular modeling. *Biochemistry, 34*(33), 10365–10375.

Miners, J. O., Coulter, S., Tukey, R. H., Veronese, M. E., & Birkett, D. J. (1996). Cytochromes P450, 1A2, and 2C9 are responsible for the human hepatic O-demethylation of R- and S-naproxen. *Biochemical Pharmacology, 51*(8), 1003–1008.

Mizutani, T. (2003). PM frequencies of major CYPs in Asians and Caucasians. *Drug Metabolism Reviews, 35*(2 & 3), 99–106.

Murphy, A., & Wilbur, K. (2003). Phenytoin-diazepam interaction. *Annals of Pharmacotherapy, 37*(5), 659–663.

O'Donnell, J. P., Dalvie, D. K., Kalgutkar, A. S., & Obach, R. S. (2003). Mechanism-based inactivation of human recombinant P450 2C9 by the nonsteroidal anti-inflammatory drug suprofen. *Drug Metabolism & Disposition, 31*(11), 1369–1377.

Perini, J. A., Vianna-Jorge, R., Brogliato, A. R., & Suarez-Kurtz, G. (2005). Influence of CYP2C9 genotypes on the pharmacokinetics and pharmacodynamics of piroxicam. *Clinical Pharmacology & Therapeutics*, 78(4), 362–369.

Rodrigues, A. D. (2005). Impact of CYP2C9 genotype on pharmacokinetics: are all cyclooxygenase inhibitors the same? *Drug Metabolism & Disposition*, 33(11), 1567–1575.

Seng, K. C., Gin, G. G., Sangkar, J. V., & Phipps, M. E. (2003). Frequency of cytochrome P450 2C9 (CYP2C9) alleles in three ethnic groups in Malaysia. *Asia Pacific Journal of Molecular Biology and Biotechnology*, 11(2), 83–91.

Shintani, M., Ieiri, I., Inoue, K., Mamiya, K., Ninomiya, H., Tashiro, N., et al. (2001). Genetic polymorphisms and functional characterization of the 5'-flanking region of the human CYP2C9 gene: in vitro and in vivo studies. *Clinical Pharmacology and Therapeutics*, 70(2), 175–182.

Si, D., Guo, Y., Zhang, Y., Yang, L., Zhou, H. H., & Zhong, D. (2004). Identification of a novel variant CYP2C9 allele in Chinese. *Pharmacogenetics*, 14(7), 465–469.

Suarez-Kurtz, G. (2005). Pharmacogenomics in admixed populations. *Trends in Pharmacological Sciences*, 26(4), 196–201.

Veenstra, D. L., Blough, D. K., Higashi, M. K., Farin, F. M., Srinouanprachan, S., Rieder, M. J., & Rettie, A. E. (2005). CYP2C9 haplotype structure in European American warfarin patients and association with clinical outcomes. *Clinical Pharmacology & Therapeutics*, 77(5), 353–364.

Xie, H. G., Kim, R. B., Wood, A. J., & Stein, C. M. (2001). Molecular basis of ethnic differences in drug disposition and response. *Annual Review of Pharmacology and Toxicology*, 41, 815–850.

Xie, H.-G., Prasad, H., Kim, R., & Stein, C. M. (2002). CYP2C9 allelic variants: ethnic distribution and functional significance. *Advanced Drug Delivery Review*, 54, 1257–1270.

Yasar, U., Tybring, G., Hidestrand, M., Oscarson, M., Ingelman-Sundberg, M., Dahl, M. L., & Eliasson, E. (2001). Role of CYP2C9 polymorphism in losartan oxidation. *Drug Metabolism and Disposition*, 29(7), 1051–1056.

Zhang, Y., Zhong, D., Si, D., Guo, Y., Chen, X., & Zhou, H. (2005). Lornoxicam pharmacokinetics in relation to cytochrome P450 2C9 genotype. *British Journal of Clinical Pharmacology*, 59(1), 14–17.

WEBSITES

Karolinska Institute: Human Cytochrome P450 (*CYP*) Allele Nomenclature Committee   http://www.cypalleles.ki.se/

7

THE CYTOCHROME P450 1A2 GENE

The cytochrome P450 1A2 gene (CYP1A2) was originally described as the phenacetin-O-deethylase gene (Butler et al., 1989). This name was chosen because the enzyme produced by this gene was involved in the metabolism of an analgesic known as phenacetin. Phenacetin was discovered in 1887 and, for almost a hundred years, was widely used. It is now no longer produced because of its relatively rare, but quite serious, side effects that included hemolysis and nephropathy. The O-deethylation of phenacetin results in the production of acetaminophen, which is most widely recognized in the United States by its trade name, Tylenol (Devonshire et al., 1983). Acetaminophen is known as Paracetamol in Europe.

Because phenacetin is no longer produced, the original name of this gene, phenacetin O-deethylase, is now an anachronism in the same way that the original name for the CYP2D6 gene (i.e., the debrisoquine hydroxylase gene) is an anachronism. Since neither phenacetin nor debrisoquine is used in practice, their original names convey little relevant meaning. Like the debrisoquine hydroxylase enzyme, the phenacetin O-deethylase enzyme is a member of the P450 family of enzymes. Consequently, phenacetin O-deethylase has been renamed using the P450 nomenclature and is now routinely referred to as the cytochrome P450 1A2 enzyme or more simply as the 1A2 enzyme.

Until it was banned in the United States in 1983, phenacetin was included in a popular over-the-counter preparation composed of aspirin, phenacetin, and caffeine that had the nickname "APC" and was widely taken as a "pick-me-up" or as a "pain killer." There was no appreciation at the time that differential capacity to metabolize phenacetin could be the result of genetic variability in the CYP1A2 gene. Consequently, it was not appreciated that poor metabolizers were at increased risk of developing adverse effects, such as anemia and kidney disease. Given that both phenacetin and caffeine are metabolized by CYP1A2, poor metabolizers of CYP1A2 were at particularly high risk for adverse responses to this compound.

Over 40 currently available drugs are primarily metabolized by the 1A2 enzyme. These include some commonly prescribed psychotropic medications. The 1A2 enzyme also plays an important secondary role in the metabolism of other psychotropic drugs when their primary pathways are not functional.

LOCATION AND GENE VARIATION

CYP1A2 is located on chromosome 15. The specific location of the gene is on the long arm of chromosome 15 at 15q24 (Fig. 7.1).

CYP1A2 consists of approximately 7,758 nucleotides or about 7.8 kilobases. It contains seven exons, which are composed of 3,127 nucleotides, and codes for a polypeptide that is composed of 516 amino acids (Fig. 7.2). The first exon is a noncoding exon. Therefore, using the Karolinska methodology, the locations of nucleotides that make up the first exon are designated using negative numbers. Significant variations have now been reported in all of the coding exons.

CYP1A2 is highly variable and this variability occurs primarily in the intronic DNA of the gene. The Karolinska Institute has catalogued the verified CYP1A2 variants on its website (http://www.cypalleles.ki.se/). Currently, 36 known variants have been catalogued into 21 allele classes. Table 7.1 lists 14 relatively common CYP1A2 variations that can be identified by clinical reference laboratories and the activity level of the enzymes produced by each of these alleles. The mean estimated allele frequency of each of these alleles in Northern European populations is also included in Table 7.1.

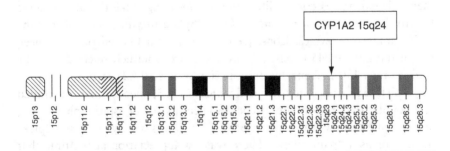

FIGURE 7.1. Chromosome 15 with arrow to designate the location of the 1A2 gene.

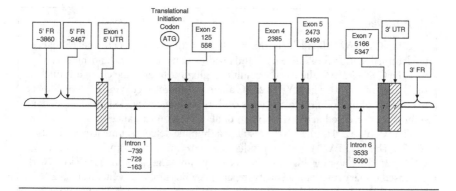

FIGURE 7.2. CYP1A2 structure illustrating the location of the 7 exons and the single nucleotide polymorphisms that define the most important 1A2 alleles.

TABLE 7.1. Activity level of the most commonly genotyped 1A2 alleles

Allele	Activity Level	Northern European Allele Frequency %
*1A	Normal	60[1]
*1B	Normal	
*1C	Variable Inducibility	
*1D	Inducible	4.8
*1F	Inducible	33[2]
*1K	Decreased	0.4
*3	Decreased	<0.1
*4	Decreased	0.5
*6	None	0.5
*7	None	<0.1
*8	Decreased	<0.1
*11	Decreased	<0.1
*15	Decreased	<0.1
*16	Decreased	<0.1

[1]Currently, the relative allele frequency of *1A, *1B, and *1C are not consistently reported and further studies are needed to differentiate the frequency of each of these three alleles.
[2]The frequency of *1F varies widely in ethnic groups, but it is reported to be between 30% and 33% in most studies of European samples.

Technical Discussion of CYP1A2 Variations (see Fig. 7.2, Tables 7.1 and 7.2)

Each of the most well-studied CYP1A2 alleles is described in this technical discussion. Although clinicians do not need to learn the precise nucleotide changes that influence CYP1A2 enzyme activity levels, the following section is presented for those who are interested in molecular genetic mechanisms.

The CYP1A2*1A allele is the wild-type or reference structure of the gene and produces an enzyme with normal activity.

(*Continued*)

The CYP1A2*1B allele is the result of a thymine to cytosine change at nucleotide location 5347 in exon 7 and produces an enzyme with normal activity.

The CYP1A2*1C allele is the result of a guanine to adenine change at nucleotide location –3860. The CYP1A2*1C allele produces an enzyme for which there is evidence of inducibility for patients of European ancestry. This allele may have somewhat decreased activity in some populations of Asian ancestry.

The CYP1A2*1D allele is the result of a thymine deletion at nucleotide location –2467. The CYP1A2*1D allele produces an enzyme which can be induced. The CYP1A2*1D polymorphism is induced by smoking and is associated with increased urinary tract mutagenicity in patients who smoke (Pavanello et al., 2007).

The CYP1A2*1F allele is the result of a cytosine to adenine change at nucleotide location –163 in intron 1. The CYP1A2*1F allele has been shown to be induced by smoking and may contribute significantly to the substantial interindividual variation in CYP1A2 activity (Sachse et al., 2003).

The CYP1A2*1K allele is defined by three SNPs in intron 1. These are a thymine-to-guanine change at nucleotide location –739, a cytosine to thymine change at nucleotide location –729, and a cytosine to adenine change at nucleotide location –163. The CYP1A2*1K allele produces an enzyme with decreased activity.

The CYP1A2*3 allele is the result of a thymine to cytosine change at nucleotide location 5347 in exon 7, which characterizes the CYP1A2*1B variant. The *3 allele also has a guanine to adenine change at nucleotide location 2385 in exon 4. CYP1A2*3 produces an enzyme with decreased activity.

The CYP1A2*4 allele is the result of an adenine to thymine change at nucleotide location 2499 in exon 5. The CYP1A2*4 allele produces an enzyme with decreased activity.

The CYP1A2*6 allele is the result of a cytosine to thymine change at nucleotide location 5090 in intron 6. The CYP1A2*6 allele produces an enzyme with no activity.

The CYP1A2*7 allele is the result of a guanine to adenine change at nucleotide location 3533 in intron 6. The CYP1A2*7 allele produces an enzyme with no activity due to a splicing defect.

The CYP1A2*8 allele is the result of a guanine to adenine change at nucleotide location 5166 in exon 7. The *8 allele also has a thymine to cytosine change at nucleotide location 5347 in exon 7, which also characterizes CYP1A2*1B, CYP1A2*3, CYP1A2*15, and CYP1A2*16. CYP1A2*8 produces an enzyme with decreased activity.

The CYP1A2*11 allele is the result of a cytosine to adenine change at nucleotide location 558 in exon 2. The CYP1A2*11 allele produces an enzyme with decreased activity.

The CYP1A2*15 allele is the result of a cytosine to guanine change at nucleotide location 125 in exon 2. The *15 allele also has a thymine to cytosine change at nucleotide location 5347 in exon 7, which characterizes CYP1A2*1B, CYP1A2*3, CYP1A2*8, and CYP1A2*16. CYP1A2*15 produces an enzyme with decreased activity.

The CYP1A2*16 allele is the result of a guanine to adenine change at nucleotide location 2473 in exon 5. The *16 allele also has a thymine to cytosine change at nucleotide location 5347 in exon 7, which characterizes the CYP1A2*1B, CYP1A2*3, CYP1A2*8, and CYP1A2*15. CYP1A2*16 produces an enzyme with decreased activity.

TABLE 7.2. CYP1A2 variations that define 14 common alleles

CYP1A2 Allele	Enzyme Activity	5'UTR		Intron 1			Exon 2		Exon 4	Exon 5		Intron 6		Exon 7	
		-3860	-2467	-739	-729	-163	125	558	2385	2473	2499	3533	5090	5166	5347
*1A	Normal	G	T	T	C	C	C	C	G	G	A	G	C	G	T
*1B	Normal	G	T	T	C	C	C	C	G	G	A	G	C	G	C
*1C	Variable Inducibility	A	T	T	C	C	C	C	G	G	A	G	C	G	T
*1D	Inducible	G	Deletion of T	T	C	C		C	G	G	A	G	C	G	T
*1F	Inducible	G	T	T	C	A	C	C	G	G	A	G	C	G	T
*1K	Decreased	G	T	G	T	A	C	C	G	G	A	G	C	G	T
*3	Decreased	G	T	T	C	C	C	C	A	G	A	G	C	G	C
*4	Decreased	G	T	T	C	C	C	C	G	G	T	G	C	G	T
*6	None	G	T	T	C	C	C	C	G	G	A	G	T	G	T
*7	None	G	T	T	C	C	C	C	G	G	A	A	C	G	T
*8	Decreased	G	T	T	C	C	C	C	G	G	A	A	C	A	C
*11	Decreased	G	T	T	C	C	C	A	G	G	A	G	C	G	T
*15	Decreased	G	T	T	C	C	G	C	G	A	A	G	C	G	C
*16	Decreased	G	T	T	C	C	C	C	G	A	A	G	C	G	C

This table documents the specific nucleotide variations that define common alleles of CYP1A2. Each row represents an allele, which is designated by a "*" with a number and letter, or a "*" with a number only. Each column represents a location on the gene map. The *1A row is the "wild-type" reference sequence. Shaded nucleotides represent variations from the wild-type reference sequence.

TABLE 7.3. Variability in allele frequencies of four geographical populations

Geographic Ancestry	*1A (%)	*1D (%)	*1F (%)	*1K (%)
Northern European	31	8	42	4
Ethiopian	40	<0.1	50	3
Sub-Saharan African	38	<0.1	51	<0.1
Japanese	<0.1	42	63	<0.1

These allele frequencies are based on multiple reports in the literature.

GENOTYPIC VARIANCE ACROSS GEOGRAPHIC ANCESTRY

Like other cytochrome P450 drug-metabolizing enzyme genes, CYP1A2 has considerable genotypic variation across different geographic ancestral groups. The ancestral groups identified in Table 7.3 illustrate this variation.

Northern Europeans

Although CYP1A2*1F is a quite common allele in Northern Europeans, it is even more common in African and Japanese populations. Although the CYP1A2*1A is quite common in Europeans, it is very rare in Japanese populations (Skarke et al., 2005).

Ethiopians

The reported allelic frequency of CYP1A2 variants in the Ethiopian population suggests that the CYP1A2*1A allele frequency is about 40%, whereas the CYP1A2*1F allele is estimated to be 50%. The frequency of the CYP1A2*1K allele is about 3%, whereas the CYP1A2*1D allele has not been reported in Ethiopians (Aklillu et al., 2003).

Sub-Saharan Africans

The CYP1A2*1F allele is the most common CYP1A2 allele in this population and has an allele frequency of about 51%. The CYP1A2*1A allele has a frequency of about 38%. The CYP1A2*1D and CYP1A2*1K alleles have not been reported in Sub-Saharan African populations (Skarke et al., 2005).

Japanese

In the Japanese population, the most common allele is the CYP1A2*1F variant and has an allele frequency of about 63%. The CYP1A2*1D is also commonly found and has an allele frequency of about 42%. The CYP1A2*1K allele has not been reported in Japanese samples (Soyama et al., 2005).

DEFINING CYP1A2 METABOLIC PHENOTYPES

Virtually all individuals have two copies of the CYP1A2 gene, which distinguishes it from CYP2D6, which has multiple duplications. Given that 14 CYP1A2 alleles can be identified, there are many possible CYP1A2 genotypes. By tradition, this variability has been made more manageable by classifying patients into the four broad clinical metabolic phenotypes as has been developed for CYP2D6 phenotype reporting. However, it is increasingly clear that some precision in estimating metabolic capacity is lost using this method.

Definition of the Poor CYP1A2 Metabolizer Phenotype

The working definition of a CYP1A2 poor metabolizer is a patient who does not have a normal CYP1A2 allele. Given that seven alleles of CYP1A2 provide good evidence that they produce an enzyme with decreased activity, there are many possible combinations of decreased activity alleles.

Definition of the Intermediate CYP1A2 Metabolizer Phenotype

The definition of an intermediate CYP1A2 phenotype is a patient who has only one fully active allele and one allele that produces an enzyme with decreased activity. There are two well-studied active forms of CYP1A2, which are distinguished by their inducibility. The CYP1A2*1A allele is not easily inducible, whereas the CYP1A2*1F allele is highly inducible. Consequently, in the absence of an inducer, the activities of the CYP1A2*1A allele and the CYP1A2*1F allele are similar. However, if an inducer is present, the activity of CYP1A2*1F increases, as does the activity of CYP1A2*1C in patients of European ancestry.

CYP1A2 Extensive Metabolizer Phenotype

Patients are designated as having the extensive metabolizer phenotype if they have either the *1A/*1A genotype or the *1A/*1F genotype. Patients with the *1A/*1A genotype will have a lower level of enzyme activity than patients with the *1A/*1F genotype when they are exposed to an inducer.

TABLE 7.4. Inducers of CYP1A2

CYP1A2 Inducers	Relevant Comments
Tobacco	Smoking is the most common CYP1A2 inducer.
Insulin	Insulin is a peptide hormone produced in the islets of Langerhan in the pancreas and used in the treatment of diabetes (Melkersson et al., 2007).
Modafinil	Modafinil is used to treat narcolepsy.
Nafcillin	Nafcillin is a semisynthetic penicillin analogue that is effective against penicillinase-producing *Staphylococcus aureus*.
Omeprazole	Omeprazole is a proton-pump inhibitor used in the treatment of peptic ulcer disease (Han et al., 2002).
Cruciferous Vegetables	Cruciferous vegetables include such vegetables as Brussels sprouts, broccoli, cabbage, and watercress.

CYP1A2 Ultra-Rapid Metabolizer Phenotype

The *1D/*1D, *1D/*1F and *1F/*1F genotypes predict ultra-rapid CYP1A2 metabolism, but the ultra-rapid phenotype is only expressed in the presence of enzyme induction. The *1C/*1C, *1C/*1D and *1C/*1F genotypes in patients of European ancestry also predict ultra-rapid phenotype, but these genotypes have not been demonstrated to predict the ultra-rapid phenotype in patients who are not of European ancestry. Consequently, when CYP1A2 medications are prescribed, there should be careful clinical monitoring of patient exposure to CYP1A2 inducers, which are listed in Table 7.4. Further research is needed to clarify if other alleles of CYP1A2 may also be inducible.

ANTIDEPRESSANT MEDICATIONS

Fluvoxamine is the only antidepressant metabolized primarily by the CYP1A2 enzyme. Additionally, duloxetine, clomipramine, and imipramine are substantially metabolized by the CYP1A2 enzyme. Mirtazapine and amitriptyline are minimally metabolized by CYP1A2, but the CYP1A2 genotype may be important for the metabolism of these antidepressants if their primary enzymes are inactive (Table 7.5).

Fluvoxamine

Fluvoxamine is a selective serotonin reuptake inhibitor antidepressant. Fluvoxamine has no active metabolites and is primarily metabolized by CYP1A2. Fluvoxamine also inhibits the CYP1A2 enzyme.

TABLE 7.5. Antidepressant medications metabolized by the 1A2 enzyme

Antidepressants Primarily Metabolized by 1A2	Antidepressants Substantially Metabolized by 1A2	Antidepressants Minimally Metabolized by 1A2
Fluvoxamine	Duloxetine Clomipramine Imipramine	Mirtazapine Amitriptyline

Duloxetine

Duloxetine is an antidepressant that blocks the reuptake of serotonin and norepinephrine. It has also been reported to have an analgesic effect in patients with pain related to diabetic peripheral neuropathy. In addition to CYP1A2, CYP2D6 plays a role in the metabolism of duloxetine. To a lesser extent, duloxetine blocks reuptake of dopamine at the receptors.

Clomipramine

Clomipramine is a tricyclic antidepressant that has been widely used for the treatment of obsessive-compulsive symptoms. In addition to CYP1A2, clomipramine is metabolized by CYP2C19, CYP3A4, and CYP2D6 (Nielsen et al., 1996).

Imipramine

Imipramine is a tertiary amine tricyclic antidepressant that is used to treat depression and enuresis. Imipramine inhibits the reuptake of serotonin more than most secondary amine tricyclics, as it blocks the reuptake of serotonin and norepinephrine almost equally. Imipramine also has substantial activity at the D_1 and D_2 dopamine receptors.

Imipramine is primarily metabolized by CYP1A2, CYP2C19, and CYP3A4 to its active metabolite desipramine by N-demethylation. Imipramine is also hydroxylated to 2-hydroxy-imipramine by CYP2D6. In patients who are poor 2D6 metabolizers, this hydroxylation can be facilitated by CYP2C19. Drugs that inhibit CYP2D6 result in an increase in the serum concentration of both imipramine and desipramine (Linnet, 2004).

Mirtazapine

Mirtazapine is an antidepressant with a tetracyclic chemical structure that enhances both noradrenergic and serotonergic neurotransmission. In addition to CYP1A2, mirtazapine is metabolized by CYP2D6 and CYP3A4 (Anttila & Leinonen, 2001).

Amitriptyline

Amitriptyline is a tricyclic antidepressant that inhibits serotonin and noradrenaline reuptake almost equally. The major metabolic pathway for amitriptyline is demethylation, which is catalyzed by CYP2C19 and results in the active metabolite, nortriptyline. Alternative minor pathways for the metabolism of amitriptyline are hydroxylation by CYP2D6 and demethylation by CYP1A2, CYP2C9, and CYP3A4 (Steimer et al., 2004).

Antipsychotic Medications

Clozapine and olanzapine are predominantly metabolized by the CYP1A2 enzyme. Chlorpromazine is substantially metabolized by the CYP1A2 enzyme. Thioridazine and haloperidol are minimally metabolized by CYP1A2 (Table 7.6).

Clozapine

Clozapine was the first atypical antipsychotic and has one major metabolite, which is also pharmacologically active. CYP1A2 is primarily responsible for clozapine metabolism. However, CYP2C19, CYP2D6, CYP2E1, CYP3A4, and CYP3A5 can provide alternative metabolic pathways (Linnet & Olesen, 1997).

Olanzapine

Olanzapine is an atypical antipsychotic that is primarily metabolized by CYP1A2 and secondarily metabolized by CYP2D6.

Chlorpromazine

Chlorpromazine was the first phenothiazine used to treat psychotic patients, and has minimal effect on the serotonergic pathways. It is metabolized by both CYP1A2 and CYP2D6.

Table 7.6. Antipsychotic medications metabolized by the 2D6 enzyme

Antipsychotic Medications Predominantly Metabolized by CYP1A2	Antipsychotic Medications Substantially Metabolized by CYP1A2	Antipsychotic Medications Minimally Metabolized by CYP1A2
Clozapine Olanzapine	Chlorpromazine	Thioridazine Haloperidol

Haloperidol

Haloperidol is a typical antipsychotic drug. It is a butyrophenone, but produces pharmacological effects similar to those of the phenothiazine antipsychotics. It is primarily metabolized by CYP3A4 and CYP2D6. However, CYP1A2 does contribute to the metabolism of haloperidol, as has been demonstrated by evaluating patients who have received a CYP1A2 inhibitor and subsequently experienced increased serum levels of haloperidol (Daniel et al., 1994).

Thioridazine

Thioridazine is a phenothiazine that is a racemic compound with two enantiomers. Both enantiomers are metabolized by CYP2D6, but CYP1A2 metabolism becomes important for patients who are taking thioridazine and who are poor 2D6 metabolizers.

OTHER CYP1A2 SUBSTRATE MEDICATIONS AND SUBSTANCES

Acetaminophen

Acetaminophen is an analgesic metabolized by the CYP1A2 and CYP2E1 enzymes. Given that a metabolite of acetaminophen can be toxic to the liver, ultra-rapid CYP1A2 metabolizers, who more efficiently metabolize acetaminophen, are more vulnerable to liver damage if large doses of acetaminophen are consumed.

Caffeine

Caffeine is a central nervous system stimulant that is completely absorbed within 45 minutes of ingestion. It is metabolized by the CYP1A2 enzyme into three metabolic dimethylxanthines.

Cyclobenzaprine

Cyclobenzaprine is a centrally acting skeletal muscle relaxant that is structurally related to trazodone and the first-generation tricyclic antidepressants. Cyclobenzaprine is metabolized primarily by CYP1A2, although both CYP3A4 and CYP2D6 also play a role in its metabolism.

Naproxen

Naproxen is a nonsteroidal anti-inflammatory drug (NSAID) that is metabolized by both CYP1A2 and CYP2C9. The metabolic clearance of the S-naproxen enantiomer is determined largely by the activities of these two enzymes (Miners et al., 1996).

Ondansetron

Ondansetron is a serotonin $5\text{-}HT_3$ receptor antagonist that is used as an antiemetic to treat nausea following chemotherapy. CYP2B6 plays a major role in the metabolism of ondansetron, but CYP1A2, CYP2D6, and CYP3A4 are also involved in its metabolism (Niwa et al., 2006).

Propranolol

Propranolol is a nonselective β-blocker that is metabolized by CYP1A2.

Riluzole

Riluzole is a drug used to treat amyotrophic lateral sclerosis and is primarily metabolized by the CYP1A2 enzyme (van Kan et al., 2004).

Ropivacaine

Ropivacaine is a local anaesthetic drug belonging to the amino amide group. CYP1A2 is the primary enzyme for the metabolism of ropivacaine, but CYP3A4 also plays a role (Arlander et al., 1998).

Tacrine

Tacrine is a parasympathomimetic that was the first centrally acting cholinesterase inhibitor approved for the treatment of Alzheimer disease. It is metabolized by hydroxylation to its major metabolite, which is also active. Tacrine is almost exclusively metabolized by CYP1A2, which has resulted in its being used as a probe substrate to assess CYP1A2 activity (Spaldin et al., 1995).

Theophylline

Theophylline is a methylxanthine that has been used to treat respiratory diseases and is metabolized extensively by CYP1A2. As a xanthine, it is structurally and pharmacologically similar to caffeine.

Tizanidine

Tizanidine is a muscle relaxant and a centrally acting α2 adrenergic agonist. Concomitant use of tizanidine and moderate or potent CYP1A2 inhibitors is contraindicated. For example, the concomitant use of tizanidine and fluvoxamine has resulted in a 33-fold increase in the concentration of tizanidine, as measured by the area under the curve (AUC) in pharmacokinetic studies (Granfors et al., 2004).

Zolmitriptan

Zolmitriptan is an oral selective serotonin receptor agonist of the serotonin 1B and serotonin 1D receptors and is used in the acute treatment of migraine attacks. The metabolism of zolmitriptan is primarily dependent on CYP1A2. The monoamine oxidase-A enzyme is responsible for further metabolism of N-desmethyl-zolmitriptan, the active metabolite (Wild et al., 1999).

CLINICAL IMPLICATIONS

Patients with the *1F/*1F genotype are at increased risk for loss of efficacy of CYP1A2 substrate medication if they begin to smoke or are exposed to other inducers of CYP1A2. Poor CYP1A2 metabolizers are at increased risk for adverse reactions when taking CYP1A2 substrate medications.

Clinical Case 6

The psychotic symptoms of a 42-year-old woman with schizophrenia had been well controlled on olanzapine for 3 years. Unfortunately, she had gained 50 pounds during the course of her treatment over this time. As a result, her husband had become very critical of her appearance and threatened to leave her. She decided to go on a vegetarian diet and began smoking heavily in an attempt to lose weight. One week after beginning her diet, her psychotic symptoms returned. Subsequently, pharmacogenomic testing was ordered (Table 7.7).

TABLE 7.7. Pharmacogenomic report of case 6

Pharmacogenomic Report of Case 6		
Gene	Genotype of Patient	Clinical Implication
CYP2D6	*1/*2A	Extensive CYP2D6 metabolizer
CYP2C19	*1/*1	Extensive CYP2C19 metabolizer
CYP2C9	*1/*2	Intermediate CYP2C9 metabolizer
CYP1A2	*1F/*1F	Ultra-rapid CYP1A2 metabolizer (when exposed to induction)

(*Continued*)

This patient is a CYP1A2 ultra-rapid metabolizer when a CYP1A2 inducer is present. The combination of smoking and consuming large amounts of cruciferous vegetables rapidly induced the metabolism of the olanzapine that she was taking. This resulted in a rapid decrease in her serum level and the relapse of her psychotic symptoms.

KEY CLINICAL CONSIDERATIONS

- Adverse side effects are more likely to occur in patients who are poor CYP1A2 metabolizers and are taking CYP1A2 substrate medications.
- Induction of patients with the ultra-rapid CYP1A2 phenotype can lead to the loss of the therapeutic effect of CYP1A2 substrate medications. This has been commonly observed in patients with schizophrenia who are treated with clozapine or olanzapine in an inpatient facility that does not allow smoking. On discharge, when the patient resumes smoking, the loss of therapeutic efficacy can be quite rapid.

REFERENCES

Aklillu, E., Carrillo, J. A., Makonnen, E., Hellman, K., Pitarque, M., Bertilsson, L., et al. (2003). Genetic polymorphism of CYP1A2 in Ethiopians affecting induction and expression: characterization of novel haplotypes with single-nucleotide polymorphisms in intron 1. *Molecular Pharmacology, 64*(3), 659–669.

Anttila, S. A., & Leinonen, E. V. (2001). A review of the pharmacological and clinical profile of mirtazapine. *CNS Drug Reviews, 7*(3), 249–264.

Arlander, E., Ekstrom, G., Alm, C., Carrillo, J. A., Bielenstein, M., Bottiger, Y., et al. (1998). Metabolism of ropivacaine in humans is mediated by CYP1A2 and to a minor extent by CYP3A4: an interaction study with fluvoxamine and ketoconazole as in vivo inhibitors. *Clinical Pharmacology & Therapeutics, 64*(5), 484–491.

Butler, M. A., Iwasaki, M., Guengerich, F. P., & Kadlubar, F. F. (1989). Human cytochrome P-450PA (P-450IA2), the phenacetin O-deethylase, is primarily responsible for the hepatic 3-demethylation of caffeine and N-oxidation of carcinogenic arylamines. *Proceedings of the National Academy of Sciences of the United States of America, 86*(20), 7696–7700.

Daniel, D. G., Randolph, C., Jaskiw, G., Handel, S., Williams, T., Abi-Dargham, A., et al. (1994). Coadministration of fluvoxamine increases serum concentrations of haloperidol. *Journal of Clinical Psychopharmacology, 14*(5), 340–343.

Devonshire, H. W., Kong, I., Cooper, M., Sloan, T. P., Idle, J. R., & Smith, R. L. (1983). The contribution of genetically determined oxidation status to inter-individual variation in phenacetin disposition. *British Journal of Clinical Pharmacology*, 16(2), 157–166.

Granfors, M. T., Backman, J. T., Neuvonen, M., & Neuvonen, P. J. (2004). Ciprofloxacin greatly increases concentrations and hypotensive effect of tizanidine by inhibiting its cytochrome P450 1A2-mediated presystemic metabolism. *Clinical Pharmacology & Therapeutics*, 76(6), 598–606.

Han, X. M., Ouyang, D. S., Chen, X. P., Shu, Y., Jiang, C. H., Tan, Z. R., et al. (2002). Inducibility of CYP1A2 by omeprazole in vivo related to the genetic polymorphism of CYP1A2. *British Journal of Clinical Pharmacology*, 54(5), 540–543.

Linnet, K. (2004). In vitro microsomal metabolism of imipramine under conditions mimicking the in vivo steady-state situation. *Human Psychopharmacology*, 19(1), 31–36.

Linnet, K., & Olesen, O. V. (1997). Metabolism of clozapine by cDNA-expressed human cytochrome P450 enzymes. *Drug Metabolism & Disposition*, 25(12), 1379–1382.

Melkersson, K. I., Scordo, M. G., Gunes, A., & Dahl, M. L. (2007). Impact of CYP1A2 and CYP2D6 polymorphisms on drug metabolism and on insulin and lipid elevations and insulin resistance in clozapinetreated patients. *The Journal of clinical psychiatry*, 68(5), 697–704.

Miners, J. O., Coulter, S., Tukey, R. H., Veronese, M. E., & Birkett, D. J. (1996). Cytochromes P450, 1A2, and 2C9 are responsible for the human hepatic O-demethylation of R- and S-naproxen. *Biochemical Pharmacology*, 51(8), 1003–1008.

Nielsen, K. K., Flinois, J. P., Beaune, P., & Brosen, K. (1996). The biotransformation of clomipramine in vitro, identification of the cytochrome P450s responsible for the separate Metabolic Pathways. *The Journal of Pharmacology and Experimental Therapeutics*, 277(3), 1659–1664.

Niwa, T., Yamamoto, S., Saito, M., Kobayashi, N., Ikeda, K., Noda, Y., & Takagi, A. (2006). Effects of serotonin-3 receptor antagonists on cytochrome P450 activities in human liver microsomes. *Biological & Pharmaceutical Bulletin*, 29(9), 1931–1935.

Pavanello, S., B'Chir, F., Pulliero, A., Saguem, S., Ben Fraj, R., El Aziz Hayouni, A., et al. (2007). Interaction between CYP1A2-T2467DELT polymorphism and smoking in adenocarcinoma and squamous cell carcinoma of the lung. *Lung Cancer*, 57(3), 266–272.

Sachse, C., Bhambra, U., Smith, G., Lightfoot, T. J., Barrett, J. H., Scollay, J., et al. & Colorectal Cancer Study, G. (2003). Polymorphisms in the cytochrome P450 CYP1A2 gene (CYP1A2) in colorectal cancer patients and controls: allele frequencies, linkage disequilibrium and influence on caffeine metabolism. *British Journal of Clinical Pharmacology*, 55(1), 68–76.

Skarke, C., Kirchhof, A., Geisslinger, G., & Lotsch, J. (2005). Rapid genotyping for relevant CYP1A2 alleles by pyrosequencing. *European Journal of Clinical Pharmacology*, 61(12), 887–892.

Soyama, A., Saito, Y., Hanioka, N., Maekawa, K., Komamura, K., Kamakura, S., et al. (2005). Single nucleotide polymorphisms and haplotypes of CYP1A2 in a Japanese population. [erratum appears in *Drug Metab Pharmacokinet* 2005;20(2):152]. *Drug Metabolism & Pharmacokinetics, 20*(1), 24–33.

Spaldin, V., Madden, S., Adams, D. A., Edwards, R. J., Davies, D. S., & Park, B. K. (1995). Determination of human hepatic cytochrome P4501A2 activity in vitro use of tacrine as an isoenzyme-specific probe. *Drug Metabolism & Disposition, 23*(9), 929–934.

Steimer, W., Zopf, K., Von Amelunxen, S., Pfeiffer, H., Bachofer, J., Popp, J., et al. (2004). Allele-specific change of concentration and functional gene dose for the prediction of steady-state serum concentrations of amitriptyline and nortriptyline in CYP2C19 and CY2D6 extensive and intermediate metabolizers. *Clinical Chemistry, 50*(9), 1623–1633.

van Kan, H. J., Groeneveld, G. J., Kalmijn, S., Spieksma, M., van den Berg, L. H., & Guchelaar, H. J. (2004). Association between CYP1A2 activity and riluzole clearance in patients with amyotrophic lateral sclerosis. *British Journal of Clinical Pharmacology, 59*(3), 310–313.

Wild, M. J., McKillop, D., & Butters, C. J. (1999). Determination of the human cytochrome P450 isoforms involved in the metabolism of zolmitriptan. *Xenobiotica, 29*(8), 847–857.

WEBSITES

Karolinska Institute: Human Cytochrome P450 (*CYP*) Allele Nomenclature Committee   http://www.cypalleles.ki.se/

III

A GENE ASSOCIATED WITH THE METABOLISM OF NEUROTRANSMITTERS

8

THE CATECHOL-O-METHYLTRANSFERASE GENE

The catechol-O-methyltransferase (COMT) enzyme is responsible for the O-methylation of catecholamines, which are chemical compounds derived from the amino acid tyrosine (Axelrod & Tomchick, 1958). Although the structural organization of COMT is currently conceptualized as a single gene, this single gene codes for two similar enzymes. One is soluble and is referred to as S-COMT. The other is membrane-bound and is referred to as MB-COMT.

The COMT enzyme inactivates circulating catechol neurotransmitters through the process of methylation. COMT also inactivates L-dopa, a catechol-containing drug that is a dopamine precursor used in the treatment of Parkinson disease (Dousa et al., 2003; Mannisto & Kaakkola, 1999; Tenhunen et al., 1994).

A well-known genetic variation of COMT was described more than 30 years ago (Weinshilboum & Raymond, 1977). This genetic variation has been referred to for many years as the Val158Met polymorphism, referring to the amino acid change at position 158 in the amino acid sequence of the membrane-bound form of the enzyme. It has also been less commonly referred to as 472G/A. This functional polymorphism has now been assigned a unique reference sequence number, which is rs4680. The Val allele (i.e., guanine allele) of rs4680 is a more active allele than the Met allele (i.e., adenine allele) and has been considered a risk factor for schizophrenia (Chen et al., 2004).

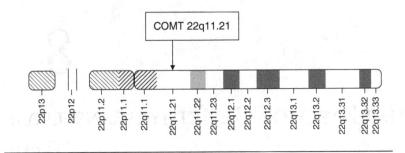

FIGURE 8.1. Chromosome 22 with arrow to designate the location of COMT.

LOCATION AND GENE VARIATION

The COMT gene is located on chromosome 22, which is the shortest auto-some. The specific location of COMT is on the long arm of chromosome 22 at 22q11.21 (Fig. 8.1).

COMT consists of 27,222 nucleotides or 27.2 kilobases. It contains six exons, which are composed of 1,290 nucleotides and codes for a

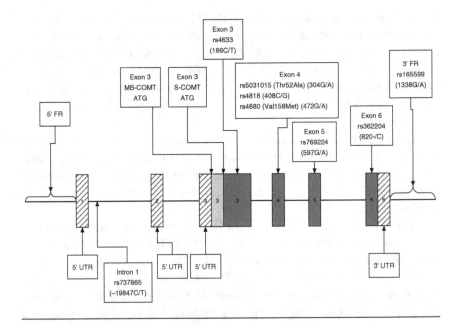

FIGURE 8.2. The structure of COMT illustrating the location of the six exons and the single nucleotide polymorphisms that define the most important COMT alleles.

The 3' portion of this entire gene codes for the S-COMT enzyme. Tenhunen et al. (1994).

polypeptide composed of either 221 or 271 amino acids. Its soluble enzyme (S-COMT) contains 221 amino acids. Its membrane-bound enzyme (MB-COMT) contains an additional 50 amino acids, resulting in a total of 271 amino acids (Mannisto & Kaakkola, 1999) (Fig. 8.2).

Exon 1 and exon 2 of COMT are noncoding exons. The expression of COMT is controlled by two distinct promoters. Both promoters are located in exon 3. The distal promoter (P2) regulates synthesis of a 1.5-kb mRNA species. The mRNA regulated by the P2 promoter can code for both the MB-COMT and S-COMT proteins. The expression of a shorter transcript (1.3 kb) is regulated by the P1 promoter. The P1 promoter is located between the S-COMT ATG start codon and the MB-COMT ATG start codon (Mannisto & Kaakkola, 1999).

The S-COMT enzyme does not play a major role in the regulation of the central nervous system (CNS). However, the MB-COMT enzyme catalyzes O-methylation in the brain and contributes to the metabolism of endogenous catecholamines that are present in the CNS (Bertocci et al., 1991). The MB-COMT enzyme is also located in the erythrocytes and the liver. MB-COMT is an integral membrane protein that is structurally distinct from the cytosolic S-COMT. Although both forms of COMT catalyze the O-methylation of catecholamines, the MB-COMT enzyme has a higher affinity for its substrates.

Technical Discussion of COMT Variations

Each of the most well-studied COMT alleles is described in this technical discussion.

rs737865 or −19847C/T or the Intronic Variant Sequence 1 (IVS 1)

rs737865 is the result of a cytosine to thymine change that occurs at nucleotide location −19848 in intron 1. rs737865 may be in linkage disequilibrium with a Hind III SNP, which is located upstream and is within the P2 promoter. Consequently, rs737865 may be a good surrogate marker for other variations within the P2 promoter. It is the P2 promoter that drives transcription of the MB-COMT (Palmatier et al., 2004).

rs4633 or 186C/T

rs4633 is the result of a cytosine to thymine change at nucleotide location 186 in exon 3. It is a silent mutation, as it results in anonymous change in the codon.

rs5031015 or 304G/A or Thr52/Ala

rs5031015 is the result of a guanine to adenine change at nucleotide location 304 in exon 4. rs5031015 is believed to have no significant change in the level of COMT activity. The thermal stability of the enzyme coded by the guanine allele

(*Continued*)

(i.e., the threonine allele) does not differ from that of the wild-type enzyme (Shield et al., 2004).

rs4818 or 408C/G

rs4818 is the result of a cytosine to guanine change at nucleotide location 408 in exon 4. This SNP results in anonymous change at amino acid position 136.

rs4680 or 472G/A or Val158Met

rs4680 (i.e., Val158Met) is the most well-studied COMT genetic variant. This variation is the result of a guanine to adenine change at nucleotide location 472 in exon 4. This change results in an amino acid change from valine to methionine at codon 158 of MB-COMT and at codon 108 of S-COMT. This change decreases the activity level of COMT enzyme by three- to fourfold. The change to an adenine at this location creates a polymorphic *Nla*III restriction site. The guanine allele (i.e., valine allele) is also referred to as the COMT*H allele because this allele produces a more thermostable, high-activity enzyme. The adenine allele (i.e., methionine allele) is also referred to as the COMT*L allele because this allele encodes for an enzyme with lower activity that is less thermostable.

rs769224 or 597G/A

rs769224 is the result of a guanine to adenine change at nucleotide location 597 in exon 5. It does not change the amino acid sequence, but it does obliterate an *Msp*I restriction site. The codon that includes rs769224 codes for proline at amino acid position 199 of the protein.

rs362204 or 820–/C

rs362204 is the result of the insertion of a cytosine at nucleotide location 820 in exon 6. The insertion of this cytosine alters a *Bgl*I restriction site at this location. Digestion using the restriction enzyme *Bgl*I yields either two fragments of 196 bp and 82 bp when the restriction site is present or an uncut sequence of 278 bp when the restriction site is absent.

rs165599 or 1338G/A

rs165599 at nucleotide location 1338 in the 3' flanking region (3' FR) is the result of a guanine to adenine change. A significant association between the 5' rs737865 and 3' rs165599 has been reported in schizophrenia (Shifman et al., 2002). The weak associations between rs4680 (i.e., Val158Met) and schizophrenia may be due to linkage disequilibrium with rs165599.

TABLE 8.1. Ancestral and variant alleles of some of the most commonly genotyped COMT alleles

Allele	Ancestral Allele	Variant Allele
rs737865 (−19847C/T)	C	T
rs4633 (186C/T)	C	T
rs5031015 (304G/A, Thr52Ala)	G	A
rs4818 (408C/G)	C	G
rs4680 (472G/A, Val158Met)	G	A
rs769224 (597G/A)	G	A
rs362204 (820–/C)	Deletion	C
rs165599 (1338G/A)	G	A

Mukherjee et al. (2008).

ANCESTRAL ALLELES

Table 8.1 identifies the ancestral alleles of the more common COMT single nucleotide polymorphisms (Mukherjee et al., 2008). Variations of these alleles have provided insights into the evolutionary process.

GENOTYPIC VARIANCE ACROSS GEOGRAPHIC ANCESTRY

The genetic variability of rs4680 has been widely studied in groups of different geographic ancestry (Chen et al., 1997; Li et al., 1996) (Table 8.2).

TABLE 8.2. The allele frequency of the COMT adenine or Met allele in populations with different geographic ancestry

Geographic Ancestry	Allele Frequency of the COMT Met Allele (i.e., adenine allele) (%)
Europe and Southwest Asia	47
North and Central America	34
China	27–32
Africa	23
Africa and South America	18
East Asia	24

ANTIDEPRESSANT MEDICATIONS

Bupropion

Bupropion is an atypical antidepressant that acts as both a norepinephrine and dopamine reuptake inhibitor. Bupropion is also a nicotinic antagonist. Although bupropion was initially developed as an antidepressant, it subsequently has been used to facilitate smoking cessation. Nicotine is hypothesized to induce addiction through a mechanism that results in the release of dopamine. Patients with the higher activity Val allele (i.e., the guanine allele) of rs4680 may be at a greater risk for smoking relapse when treated with bupropion, which inhibits the reuptake of dopamine (Berrettini et al., 2007).

COMT haplotypes composed of rs737865 and rs165599 have been reported to predict the efficacy of bupropion when compared with placebo. Subjects of European ancestry who had the guanine allele at both rs737865 and rs165599 did not benefit as much from bupropion treatment as did subjects with other haplotypes (Berrettini et al., 2007).

ELECTROCONVULSIVE THERAPY

Electroconvulsive therapy is a somatic treatment for major depression. Patients who are homozygous for the Val allele (i.e., guanine allele) of rs4680 have been reported to have a better response to electroconvulsive therapy than patients with other genotypes (Anttila et al., 2007).

ANTIPSYCHOTIC MEDICATIONS

Recent studies support the hypothesis that the COMT variation is related to the severity of psychotic symptomatology of schizophrenia and may have some influence on the response of patients to neuroleptic treatment (Chen et al., 2004; Molero et al., 2007).

Typical Antipsychotic Medications

A Finnish study examined the association between COMT variation and response to typical antipsychotic medications in hospitalized schizophrenic patients (Illi et al., 2003). The patients were classified as having low COMT activity or high COMT activity based on their COMT rs4680 genotypes. Patients who were homozygous for the Met allele (i.e., adenine allele) of rs4680 were classified as having "low COMT activity" as compared to patients who were heterozygous for the Met allele and Val allele or homozygous for the Val allele (i.e., guanine allele), who were classified as "high COMT activity." Patients with the low COMT activity genotype did not respond as well to typical antipsychotic medications as those with high COMT activity genotypes. A proposed explanation for this finding was that severely ill schizophrenic patients might respond less well to typical antipsychotic medication if their ability to metabolize dopamine is less effective.

Olanzapine

Olanzapine is an atypical antipsychotic that is structurally similar to clozapine. However, olanzapine has a higher affinity for 5-HT2 serotonin receptors than D2 dopamine receptors. A recent study reported that treatment with olanzapine differentially enhances working memory performance and related dorsolateral prefrontal cortex efficiency in patients, based on the COMT genotype. Patients who were homozygous for the Met allele (i.e., adenine allele) showed the greatest improvements. Patients who were heterozygous had intermediate improvements. Patients who were homozygous for the Val allele (i.e., guanine allele) had minimal improvements (Bertolino et al., 2004).

Risperidone

Risperidone is an atypical antipsychotic medication that is a selective monoaminergic antagonist and has a strong affinity for serotonin type 2 receptors and a slightly weaker affinity for dopamine type 2 receptors. A small study of Japanese schizophrenic patients treated with risperidone did not find an association between COMT genotype and response to risperidone (Yamanouchi et al., 2003).

ADVERSE EFFECTS OF ANTIPSYCHOTIC MEDICATIONS

Tardive Dyskinesia and Extrapyramidal Side Effects

In a sample from Northern India, subjects who were homozygous for the guanine allele (i.e., 408C/G) of rs4818 in exon 4 of COMT were reported to have a decreased risk of tardive dyskinesia (Srivastava et al., 2006). In this same sample, subjects who were homozygous for the Val allele (i.e., guanine allele) of rs4680 were found to be more likely to develop tardive dyskinesia.

Three other studies designed to demonstrate an association between the Val allele (i.e., guanine allele) of rs4680 and tardive dyskinesia did not demonstrate the relationship in a Turkish sample (Herken et al., 2003), a Chinese sample (Lai et al., 2005), or a Japanese sample (Matusumoto et al., 2004).

OTHER MEDICATIONS

Methylphenidate

The Val allele (i.e., guanine allele) of rs4680 has been associated with better response to methylphenidate. Specifically, 87.2% of children who were homozygous for the Val allele genotype responded to methylphenidate, as compared to 71.2% of the children who were heterozygous. In contrast, only 58.3% of children who were homozygous for the Met allele (i.e., adenine allele) responded to methylphenidate (Kereszturi et al., 2008).

Amphetamines

Studies have consistently supported the finding that subjects who are homozygous for the Val allele (i.e., guanine allele) of rs4680 respond more favorably to amphetamines (Mattay et al., 2003). This is believed to be the result of these subjects having lower baseline CNS dopamine availability, so that stimulant medication brings their dopamine concentrations to more of an optimal level. Subjects who were homozygous for the Met allele (i.e., adenine allele) had a less optimal response, as it was hypothesized that stimulants shifted their basal dopamine levels to a higher, less than optimal, level.

Modafinil

Modafinil is a stimulant used to treat narcolepsy (Dauvilliers et al., 2002). In a Swiss study, patients who were homozygous for the Val allele (i.e., guanine allele) of rs4680 did less well than patients who were heterozygous for the Val allele and Met allele or homozygous for the Met allele (i.e., adenine allele). This was true despite the fact that patients who were homozygous for the Val allele were given a higher dose.

L-dopa

L-dopa is produced from the amino acid tyrosine by the enzyme tyrosine hydroxylase and is the precursor molecule for dopamine and norepinephrine. The decarboxylation of L-dopa results in the formation of dopamine. L-dopa is also metabolized by COMT to form the metabolite 3-O-methyldopa (Dousa et al., 2003).

L-dopa is a prodrug used to increase dopamine levels in patients with Parkinson disease. L-dopa is able to cross the blood–brain barrier, whereas dopamine does not.

Morphine

Morphine is a potent opiate analgesic drug and is the principal active agent in opium. Morphine acts directly on the CNS to relieve pain, with a specific location of action being the nucleus accumbens. Morphine is highly addictive, as both physical and psychological dependence develops rapidly. rs4680 variability may be related to the efficacy of morphine, as patients with cancer pain who were homozygous for the Val allele (i.e., guanine allele) have been reported to respond more effectively to treatment with morphine (Rakvag et al., 2005).

Clinical Case 7

A 9-year-old boy who was "small for his age" had been having increased difficulties at school. He was observed to have both hyperactive and inattentive symptoms in class and at home. His parents became convinced that he needed medication, but they had read on the Internet that stimulant medication might decrease his appetite and potentially slow his growth. Family history revealed that the boy's mother had experienced intense headaches while being treated for depression using fluoxetine when she was in college. Prior to making a decision about the selection of medication for the boy, pharmacogenomic testing was ordered (Table 8.3).

TABLE 8.3. Pharmacogenomic Report of case 7

	Pharmacogenomic Report of Case 7	
Gene	Genotype	Clinical Implication
CYP2D6	*4/*5	Poor CYP2D6 metabolizer
CYP2C19	*1/*17	Extensive CYP2C19 metabolizer
CYP2C9	*1/*1	Extensive CYP2C9 metabolizer
CYP1A2	*1A/*1A	Extensive CYP1A2 metabolizer
COMT	rs4680 G/G	Good responder to methylphenidate

In considering the options of selecting methylphenidate or atomoxetine, the pharmacogenomic report revealed important new information. Significantly, the patient had only a single copy of the 2D6 gene, and this one copy was completely inactive. While this would make it less likely that he could tolerate atomoxetine at a standard dose, if he was able to manage the probable development of side effects, he might well have an improvement in his attentional symptoms (Michelson et al., 2007). However, he had an optimal COMT rs4680 genotype for response to methylphenidate. Given this information, the parents were willing to try methylphenidate, despite their concerns about the possible side effect of appetite suppression.

CLINICAL IMPLICATIONS

A variety of pharmacogenomic predictions can be made based on variability of rs4680 (i.e.,Val158Met) variants. A potentially useful association between an rs4680 genotype and response to stimulants has been reported. Specifically, patients with higher-activity genotypes have tended to respond more reliably to methylphenidate.

KEY CLINICAL CONSIDERATIONS

- Patients who are homozygous for the Met allele (i.e., adenine allele) of rs4680 may have a higher likelihood of responding to bupropion prescribed for smoking cessation.
- Patients with schizophrenia who have the low-activity Met allele (i.e., adenine allele) of rs4680 may respond less well to typical antipsychotic medication. However, they may also have less risk of developing tardive dyskinesia.
- Patients who are homozygous for the Val allele (i.e., guanine allele) of rs4680 may have a higher likelihood of responding to methylphenidate.

REFERENCES

Anttila, S., Huuhka, K., Huuhka, M., Illi, A., Rontu, R., Leinonen, E., & Lehtimaki, T. (2007). Catechol-O-methyltransferase (COMT) polymorphisms predict treatment response in electroconvulsive therapy. *Pharmacogenomics Journal, 8*(2), 113–116.

Axelrod, J., & Tomchick, R. (1958). Enzymatic O-methylation of epinephrine and other catechols. *The Journal of Biological Chemistry, 233*(3), 702–705.

Berrettini, W. H., Wileyto, E. P., Epstein, L., Restine, S., Hawk, L., Shields, P., et al. (2007). Catechol-O-methyltransferase (COMT) gene variants predict response to bupropion therapy for tobacco dependence. *Biological Psychiatry, 61*(1), 111–118.

Bertocci, B., Miggiano, V., Da Prada, M., Dembic, Z., Lahm, H. W., & Malherbe, P. (1991). Human catechol-O-methyltransferase: cloning and expression of the membrane-associated form. *Proceedings of the National Academy of Sciences of the United States of America, 88*(4), 1416–1420.

Bertolino, A., Caforio, G., Blasi, G., De Candia, M., Latorre, V., Petruzzella, V., et al. (2004). Interaction of COMT Val108/158 Met genotype and olanzapine treatment on prefrontal cortical function in patients with schizophrenia. *American Journal of Psychiatry, 161*(10), 1798–1805.

Chen, C. H., Lee, Y. R., Wei, F. C., Koong, F. J., Hwu, H. G., & Hsiao, K. J. (1997). Association study of NlaIII and MspI genetic polymorphisms of catechol-O-methyltransferase gene and susceptibility to schizophrenia. *Biological Psychiatry, 41*, 985–987.

Chen, X., Wang, X., O'Neill, A. F., Walsh, D., & Kendler, K. S. (2004). Variants in the catechol-o-methyltransferase (COMT) gene are associated with schizophrenia in Irish high-density families. *Molecular Psychiatry, 9*(10), 962–967.

Dauvilliers, Y., Neidhart, E., Billiard, M., & Tafti, M. (2002). Sexual dimorphism of the catechol-O-methyltransferase gene in narcolepsy is associated with response to modafinil. *Pharmacogenomics Journal, 2*(1), 65–68.

Dousa, M. K., Weinshilboum, R. M., Muenter, M. D., Offord, K. P., Decker, P. A., & Tyce, G. M. (2003). L-DOPA biotransformation: correlations of dosage, erythrocyte catechol O-methyltransferase and platelet SULT1A3 activities with metabolic pathways in Parkinsonian patients. *Journal of Neural Transmission, 110*(8), 899–910.

Herken, H., Erdal, M. E., Boke, O., & Savas, H. A. (2003). Tardive dyskinesia is not associated with the polymorphisms of 5-HT2A receptor gene, serotonin transporter gene and catechol-o-methyltransferase gene. *European Psychiatry, 18*(2), 77–81.

Illi, A., Kampmanc, O., Anttilac, S., Roivasa, M., Mattilab, K., Lehtimäkib, T., & Leinonen, E. (2003). Interaction between angiotensin-converting enzyme and catechol-O-methyltransferase genotypes in schizophrenics with poor response to conventional neuroleptics. *European Neuropsychopharmacology : the journal of the European College of Neuropsychopharmacology, 13*(3), 147–151.

Kereszturi, E., Tarnok, Z., Bognar, E., Lakatos, K., Farkas, L., Gadoros, J., et al. (2008). Catechol-O-methyltransferase Val158Met polymorphism is associated with methylphenidate response in ADHD children. *American Journal of Medical Genetics Part B: Neuropsychiatric Genetics, 147B*(8), 1431–1435.

Lai, I. C., Wang, Y. C., Lin, C. C., Bai, Y. M., Liao, D. L., Yu, S. C., et al. (2005). Negative association between catechol-O-methyltransferase (COMT) gene Val158Met polymorphism and persistent tardive dyskinesia in schizophrenia. *Journal of Neural Transmission, 112*(8), 1107–1113.

Li, T., Sham, P. C., Vallada, H., Xie, T., Tang, X., Murray, R. M., et al. (1996). Preferential transmission of the high activity allele of COMT in schizophrenia. *Psychiatric Genetics, 6*, 131–133.

Mannisto, P. T., & Kaakkola, S. (1999). Catechol-O-methyltransferase (COMT): biochemistry, molecular biology, pharmacology, and clinical efficacy of the new selective COMT inhibitors. *Pharmacological Reviews, 51*(4), 593–628.

Matsumoto, C., Shinkai, T., Hori, H., Ohmori, O., & Nakamura, J. (2004). Polymorphisms of dopamine degradation enzyme (COMT and MAO) genes and tardive dyskinesia in patients with schizophrenia. *Psychiatry Research, 127*(1–2), 1–7.

Mattay, V. S., Goldberg, T. E., Fera, F., Hariri, A. R., Tessitore, A., Egan, M. F., et al. (2003). Catechol O-methyltransferase val158-met genotype and individual variation in the brain response to amphetamine. *Proceedings of* the *National Academy of Sciences of the United States of America, 100*(10), 6186–6191.

Michelson, D., Read, H. A., Ruff, D. D., Witcher, J., Zhang, S., & McCracken, J. (2007). CYP2D6 and clinical response to atomoxetine in children and adolescents with ADHD. *Journal of the American Academy of Child & Adolescent Psychiatry, 46*(2), 242–251.

Molero, P., Ortuno, F., Zalacain, M., & Patino-Garcia, A. (2007). Clinical involvement of catechol-O-methyltransferase polymorphisms in schizophrenia spectrum disorders: influence on the severity of psychotic symptoms and on the response to neuroleptic treatment. *Pharmacogenomics Journal, 7*(6), 418–426.

Mukherjee, N., Kidd, K. K., Pakstis, A. J., Speed, W. C., Li, H., Tarnok, Z., et al. (2008). The complex global pattern of genetic variation and linkage disequilibrium at catechol-O-methyltransferase. *Molecular Psychiatry*.

Palmatier, M. A., Pakstis, A. J., Speed, W., Paschou, P., Goldman, D., Odunsi, A., et al. (2004). COMT haplotypes suggest P2 promoter region relevance for schizophrenia. *Molecular Psychiatry, 9*(9), 859–870.

Rakvag, T. T., Klepstad, P., Baar, C., Kvam, T. M., Dale, O., Kaasa, S., et al. (2005). The Val158Met polymorphism of the human catechol-O-methyltransferase (COMT) gene may influence morphine requirements in cancer pain patients. *Pain, 116*(1-2), 73–78.

Shield, A. J., Thomae, B. A., Eckloff, B. W., Wieben, E. D., & Weinshilboum, R. M. (2004). Human catechol O-methyltransferase genetic variation: gene resequencing and functional characterization of variant allozymes. *Molecular Psychiatry, 9*(2), 151–160.

Shifman, S., Bronstein, M., Sternfeld, M., Pisante-Shalom, A., Lev-Lehman, E., Weizman, A., et al. (2002). A highly significant association between a COMT haplotype and schizophrenia. *American Journal of Human Genetics, 71*(6), 1296–1302.

Srivastava, V., Varma, P. G., Prasad, S., Semwal, P., Nimgaonkar, V. L., Lerer, B., et al. (2006). Genetic susceptibility to tardive dyskinesia among schizophrenia subjects: IV. Role of dopaminergic pathway gene polymorphisms. *Pharmacogenetics & Genomics, 16*(2), 111–117.

Tenhunen, J., Salminen, M., Lundstrom, K., Kiviluoto, T., Savolainen, R., & Ulmanen, I. (1994). Genomic organization of the human catechol O-methyltransferase gene and its expression from two distinct promoters. *European Journal of Biochemistry, 223*(3), 1049–1059.

Weinshilboum, R. M., & Raymond, F. A. (1977). Inheritance of low erythrocyte catechol-o-methyltransferase activity in man. *American journal of human genetics, 29*(2), 125–135.

Yamanouchi, Y., Iwata, N., Suzuki, T., Kitajima, T., Ikeda, M., & Ozaki, N. (2003). Effect of DRD2, 5-HT2A, and COMT genes on antipsychotic response to risperidone. *The Pharmacogenomics Journal, 3*, 356–361.

IV

THE NEUROTRANSMITTER
TRANSPORTER GENES

9

THE NOREPINEPHRINE TRANSPORTER GENE

The norepinephrine transporter gene (SLC6A2) is often referred to as NET or NET1. The norepinephrine transporter protein plays a role in the reuptake of norepinephrine from the synapse back into the neuron. The norepinephrine transporter also plays a secondary role in the reuptake of dopamine.

Specific antidepressant medications influence the availability of norepinephrine in the central nervous system. These antidepressants include the selective norepinephrine reuptake inhibitors (SNRIs) and the tricyclic antidepressants. The mechanism of action of cocaine and amphetamine is also believed to involve inhibition of the functioning of the norepinephrine transporter.

SLC6A2 has been studied in patients with depression, attention-deficit hyperactivity disorder (ADHD), substance abuse, Alzheimer disease, and Parkinson disease. Pharmacogenomic research designed to identify polymorphisms that predict antidepressant or antipsychotic response has been somewhat limited.

LOCATION AND GENE VARIATION

SLC6A2 is located on chromosome 16. The specific location of the gene is on the long arm of chromosome 16 at 16q12.2 (Fig. 9.1).

SLC6A2 consists of approximately 47,145 nucleotides or 47.1 kilobases. It contains 14 exons, which are composed of 3,347 nucleotides. SLC6A2 codes for a polypeptide composed of 617 amino acids (Fig. 9.2).

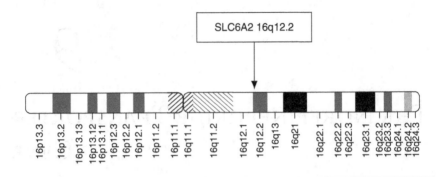

FIGURE 9.1. Chromosome 16 with arrow to designate the location of SLC6A2.

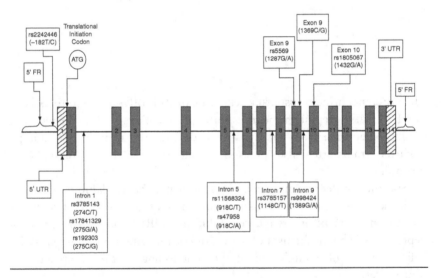

FIGURE 9.2. SLC6A2 structure illustrating the location of the 14 exons and the single nucleotide polymorphisms that define the most important SLC6A2 alleles.

Technical Discussion of SLC6A2 Variations

Each of the most well-studied SLC6A2 alleles is described in this technical discussion.

rs2242446 or –182T/C

rs2242446 (i.e., –182T/C) is the result of a thymine to cytosine change at nucleotide location –182 in the promoter region (Meary et al., 2008; Yoshida et al., 2004).

rs3785143 or 274C/T

rs3785143 (i.e., 274C/T) is the result of a cytosine to thymine change at nucleo-tide location 274 in intron 1. The thymine allele has been associated with attention-deficit hyperactivity disorder (ADHD) (Brookes et al., 2006; Kim et al., 2008).

rs17841329 or 275G/A

rs17841329 (i.e., 275G/A) is the result of a guanine to adenine change at nucleo-tide location 275 in intron 1.

rs192303 or 275C/G

rs192303 (i.e., 275C/G) is the result of a cytosine to guanine change at nucleotide location 275 in intron 1.

rs11568324 or 918C/T

rs11568324 (i.e., 918C/T) is the result of a cytosine to thymine change at nucleo-tide location 918 in intron 5. The cytosine allele has been associated with ADHD (Brookes et al., 2006; Kim et al., 2008).

rs47958 or 918C/A

rs47958 (i.e., 918C/A) is the result of a cytosine to adenine change at nucleotide location 918+498 in intron 5 (Dlugos et al., 2007).

rs3785157 or 1148C/T

rs3785157 (i.e., 1148C/T) is the result of a cytosine to thymine change at nucleo-tide location 1148 in intron 7. The thymine allele has been associated with ADHD (Bobb et al., 2005).

rs5569 or 1287G/A

rs5569 (i.e., 1287G/A) is the result of a guanine to adenine change at nucleotide location 1287 in exon 9. This change is a synonymous change, so that no change occurs in the amino acid sequence (Belfer et al., 2004; Chang et al., 2007; Meary et al., 2008; Yang et al., 2004; Zill et al., 2002).

rs (Number Unknown) 1369C/G or Ala457Pro

Ala457Pro (i.e., 1369C/G) is the result of a cytosine to a guanine change at nucleotide location 1369 in exon 9. This nucleotide change results in a change from an alanine to a proline at amino acid position 457. The cytosine allele results in a 98% loss of function compared to the guanine allele (Hahn et al., 2003; Ivancsits et al., 2003).

(*Continued*)

rs998424 or 1389G/A

rs998424 (i.e., 1389G/A) is the result of a guanine to adenine change at nucleotide location 1389 in intron 9. The cytosine allele is associated with ADHD (Bobb et al., 2005).

rs1805067 or 1432G/A

rs1805067 (i.e., 1432G/A) is the result of a guanine to adenine change at nucleotide location 1432 in exon 10 (Runkel et al., 2000). The adenine allele produces a form of the norepinephrine transporter that is three times slower at norepinephrine reuptake.

GENOTYPIC VARIANCE ACROSS GEOGRAPHIC ANCESTRY

Less extensive reporting of allele frequency is available, although there are some studies of rs2242446 and rs5569 in Asian populations.

rs2242446 or –182T/C

In a Han Chinese sample, the allele frequency of rs2242446 (i.e., –182T/C) was assessed. The allele frequency of the thymine allele was 69%, and the allele frequency of the cytosine allele was 31% (Chang et al., 2007).

In a Japanese sample, the allele frequency of rs2242446 (i.e., –182T/C) in patients with depression and in healthy volunteers was assessed (Inoue et al., 2004). In healthy subjects, the allele frequency of the thymine allele was 59%, and the allele frequency of the cytosine allele was 41%. In the depressed sample, the allele frequency of the thymine allele was 67%, and the allele frequency of the cytosine allele was 33%.

rs5569 or 1287G/A

In a Han Chinese sample, the allele frequency of rs5569 (i.e., 1287G/A) was assessed (Chang et al., 2007). The allele frequency of the guanine allele was 64%, and the allele frequency of the adenine allele was 36%.

In a Korean sample, the allele frequency of rs5569 (i.e., 1287G/A) in patients with a diagnosis of depression was assessed (Kim et al., 2006). The allele frequency of the guanine allele was 75%, and the allele frequency of the adenine allele was 25%.

ANTIDEPRESSANT MEDICATIONS

Nortriptyline

Nortriptyline is a tricyclic antidepressant that is believed to block the reuptake of norepinephrine by the norepinephrine transporter molecule. The association between variants of rs5569 (i.e., 1287G/A) and response to nortriptyline has been studied in a Korean sample. A response rate of 83% occurred in patients who were homozygous for the more common guanine allele, when compared to the response rate of 43% in patients with one or two copies of the adenine allele (Kim et al., 2006). In patients who were homozygous for the guanine allele of rs5569 and who were also homozygous for the short allele of the indel promoter polymorphism of SLC6A4, the response rate reached 89%.

Milnacipran

Milnacipran is a selective norepinephrine reuptake inhibitor that was studied in a Japanese sample with major depression. The presence of the thymine allele of rs2242446 (i.e., –182T/C) was associated with a better response to treatment with milnacipran. The presence of the guanine allele of the rs5569 (i.e., 1287G/A) polymorphism was associated with a faster response to milnacipran (Yoshida et al., 2004).

ANTIPSYCHOTIC MEDICATIONS

Risperidone and Olanzapine

A French study of patients with schizophrenia found an association between two variations of SLC6A2 and an improvement of the positive symptoms associated with schizophrenia when these patients were treated with risperidone and olanzapine (Meary et al., 2008). Patients who were homozygous for the thymine allele or heterozygous for the cytosine and thymine alleles of rs2242446 (i.e., –182T/C) demonstrated better improvement of their positive symptoms than did patients who were homozygous for the cytosine allele. Similarly, patients who were homozygous for the adenine allele of rs5569 (i.e., 1287G/A) demonstrated better improvement of positive symptoms than did patients who were heterozygous for the adenine and guanine alleles or those who were homozygous for the guanine allele.

STIMULANT MEDICATIONS

Methylphenidate

Methylphenidate consists of two isomers that are produced as a racemic mixture consisting of a d- isomer and an l- isomer. The d- isomer has strong binding affinity to both the norepinephrine transporter and the dopamine transporter, while the l- isomer has much less binding affinity to these molecules (Markowitz et al., 2006).

In a study of Han Chinese youth with ADHD, an association has been reported between a variation in rs5569 (i.e., 1287G/A) and response to methylphenidate (Yang et al., 2004). Specifically, patients who had one or two copies of the guanine allele had a symptom score reduction of 7%, whereas subjects who were homozygous for the adenine allele had a symptom score reduction of only 2% (e.g., A/A).

In a North American study of children with ADHD from various ethnic backgrounds, rs17841329 (i.e., 275G/A) and rs192303 (i.e., 275C/G) were associated with methylphenidate response. rs17841329 and rs192303 were not in linkage disequilibrium with each other (Mick et al., 2008).

Amphetamine

In a German study of healthy adults who were given a 20 mg dose of dextroamphetamine, a variant of rs47958 (i.e., 918C/A) was associated with an increased subjective sense of mood enhancement (Dlugos et al., 2007). Specifically, subjects who were homozygous for the cytosine allele achieved more elevated mood states than did subjects who had one or two copies of the adenine allele.

CLINICAL IMPLICATIONS

The clinical implications of genotyping SLC6A2 are only beginning to emerge. However, the following example highlights the potential benefit of genotyping the rs5569 variants.

Clinical Case 8

A 56-year-old Korean man presented for treatment of persistent depressive symptoms. He has been treated with both fluoxetine and venlafaxine without success. His psychiatrist ordered a pharmacogenomic profile before selecting another antidepressant (Table 9.1).

TABLE 9.1. Pharmacogenomic report of case 8

Pharmacogenomic Report of Case 8			
Gene	rs number	Genotype	Clinical Implication
CYP2D6	N/A	*2ADup/*1	Ultra-rapid CYP2D6 metabolizer
CYP2C19	N/A	*1/*1	Extensive CYP2C19 metabolizer
CYP2C9	N/A	*1/*1	Extensive CYP2C9 metabolizer
CYP1A2	N/A	*1A/*1F	Extensive CYP1A2 metabolizer
COMT	rs4680	G/G	High activity
SLC6A2	rs5569	G/G	More likely to respond to tricyclic antidepressant

Based on his SLC6A2 genotype, this patient has a high probability of having a positive response to treatment with nortriptyline (Kim et al., 2006). However, given that he is an ultra-rapid CYP2D6 metabolizer of nortriptyline, he would be unlikely to achieve an adequate serum level of this medication at recommended doses. Consequently, his serum level would need to be monitored. Given that his CYP2C19 genotype predicts that he is an extensive CYP2C19 metabolizer, he would be likely to respond to treatment with amitriptyline at a standard or moderately increased dose. The genotyping of CYP2C9, CYP1A2, and COMT did not provide any additional information that would influence his treatment.

KEY CLINICAL CONSIDERATION

- Patients who are homozygous for the guanine allele of rs5569 (i.e., 1287G/A) are more likely to respond to tricyclic antidepressants and methylphenidate than are patients who are homozygous for the adenine allele.

REFERENCES

Belfer, I., Phillips, G., Taubman, J., Hipp, H., Lipsky, R. H., Enoch, M. A., et al. (2004). Haplotype architecture of the norepinephrine transporter gene SLC6A2 in four populations. *Journal of Human Genetics, 49*(5), 232–245.

Bobb, A. J., Addington, A. M., Sidransky, E., Gornick, M. C., Lerch, J. P., Greenstein, D. K., et al. (2005). Support for association between ADHD and two candidate genes: NET1 and DRD1. *American Journal of Medical Genetics, Part B, Neuropsychiatric Genetics: The Official Publication of the International Society of Psychiatric Genetics. 134B*(1), 67–72.

Brookes, K., Xu, X., Chen, W., Zhou, K., Neale, B., Lowe, N., et al. (2006). The analysis of 51 genes in DSM-IV combined type attention deficit hyperactivity disorder: association signals in DRD4, DAT1 and 16 other genes. [erratum appears in *Mol Psychiatry*, 2006 Dec;11(12):1139 Note: Aneey, R [corrected to Anney, R]. *Molecular Psychiatry, 11*(10), 934–953.

Chang, C. C., Lu, R. B., Chen, C. L., Chu, C. M., Chang, H. A., Huang, C. C., et al. (2007). Lack of association between the norepinephrine transporter gene and major depression in a Han Chinese population. *Journal of Psychiatry & Neuroscience, 32*(2), 121–128.

Dlugos, A., Freitag, C., Hohoff, C., McDonald, J., Cook, E. H., Deckert, J., & de Wit, H. (2007). Norepinephrine transporter gene variation modulates acute response to d-Amphetamine. *Biological Psychiatry, 61*(11), 1296–1305.

Hahn, M. K., Robertson, D., & Blakely, R. D. (2003). A mutation in the human norepinephrine transporter gene (SLC6A2) associated with orthostatic intolerance disrupts surface expression of mutant and wild-type transporters. *The Journal of Neuroscience, 23*(11), 4470–4478.

Inoue, K., Itoh, K., Yoshida, K., Shimizu, T., & Suzuki, T. (2004). Positive association between T-182C polymorphism in the norepinephrine transporter gene and susceptibility to major depressive disorder in a Japanese population. *Neuropsychobiology, 50*(4), 301–304.

Ivancsits, S., Heider, A., Rudiger, H. W., & Winker, R. (2003). Orthostatic intolerance is not necessarily related to a specific mutation (Ala457Pro) in the human norepinephrine transporter gene. *American Journal of the Medical Sciences, 325*(2), 63–65.

Kim, J. W., Biederman, J., McGrath, C. L., Doyle, A. E., Mick, E., Fagerness, J., et al. (2008). Further evidence of association between two NET single-nucleotide polymorphisms with ADHD. *Molecular Psychiatry, 13*(6), 624–630.

Kim, H., Lim, S. W., Kim, S., Kim, J. W., Chang, Y. H., Carroll, B. J., & Kim, D. K. (2006). Monoamine transporter gene polymorphisms and antidepressant response in Koreans with late-life depression. *JAMA : the journal of the American Medical Association, 296*(13), 1609–1618.

Markowitz, J. S., DeVane, C. L., Pestreich, L. K., Patrick, K. S., & Muniz, R. (2006). A comprehensive in vitro screening of d-, l-, and dl-threo-methylphenidate: an exploratory study. *Journal of Child & Adolescent Psychopharmacology, 16*(6), 687–698.

Meary, A., Brousse, G., Jamain, S., Schmitt, A., Szoke, A., Schurhoff, F., et al. (2008). Pharmacogenetic study of atypical antipsychotic drug response: involvement of the norepinephrine transporter gene. *American Journal of Medical Genetics, Part B, Neuropsychiatric Genetics: the Official Publication of the International Society of Psychiatric Genetics. 147B*(4), 491–494.

Mick, E., Neale, B., Middleton, F. A., McGough, J. J., & Faraone, S. V. (2008). Genome-wide association study of response to methylphenidate in 187 children with attention-deficit/hyperactivity disorder. *American Journal of Medical Genetics. Part B, Neuropsychiatric Genetics, 147B*(8), 1412–1418.

Runkel, F., Bruss, M., Nothen, M. M., Stober, G., Propping, P., & Bonisch, H. (2000). Pharmacological properties of naturally occurring variants of the human norepinephrine transporter. *Pharmacogenetics, 10*(5), 397–405.

Yang, L., Wang, Y. F., Li, J., & Faraone, S. V. (2004). Association of norepinephrine transporter gene with methylphenidate response. *Journal of the American Academy of Child & Adolescent Psychiatry, 43*(9), 1154–1158.

Yoshida, K., Takahashi, H., Higuchi, H., Kamata, M., Ito, K., Sato, K., et al. (2004). Prediction of antidepressant response to milnacipran by norepinephrine transporter gene polymorphisms. *American Journal of Psychiatry, 161*(9), 1575–1580.

Zill, P., Engel, R., Baghai, T. C., Juckel, G., Frodl, T., Muller-Siecheneder, F., et al. (2002). Identification of a naturally occurring polymorphism in the promoter region of the norepinephrine transporter and analysis in major depression. *Neuropsychopharmacology, 26*(4), 489–493.

10

THE DOPAMINE TRANSPORTER GENE

The dopamine transporter gene (SLC6A3) is frequently referred to as DAT or DAT1. The SLC6A3 gene produces a protein that transfers dopamine from the synapse back into the neuron. Given that the process of dopamine reuptake effectively turns off the dopamine stimulation, variations in SLC6A3 have been studied in relation to psychiatric disorders such as attention-deficit hyperactivity disorder (ADHD), binge eating, depression, bipolar disorder, and alcoholism. Many promising pharmacogenomic studies have focused on the association between gene variation and response to stimulants, and there is some suggestion that, in specific patient populations, SLC6A3 variation may be associated with methylphenidate response.

LOCATION AND GENE VARIATION

SLC6A3 is located on chromosome 5. The specific location of the gene is on the short arm of chromosome 5 at 5p15.3 (Fig. 10.1).

SLC6A3 consists of approximately 52,637 nucleotides or 52.6 kilobases. It contains 15 exons, which are composed of 3,932 nucleotides. SLC6A3 codes for a polypeptide that is composed of 620 amino acids (Fig. 10.2).

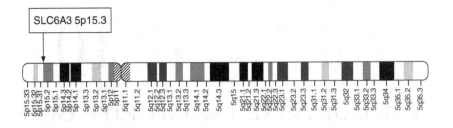

FIGURE 10.1. Chromosome 5 with arrow to designate the location of the SLC6A3 gene.

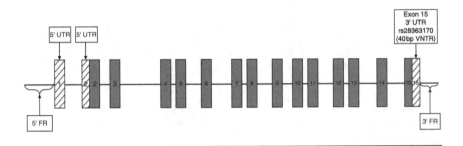

FIGURE 10.2. SLC6A3 structure illustrating the location of the 15 exons and the rs28363170 SNP in exon 15. Greenwood et al. (2002).

Technical Discussion of SLC6A3 Variations

Although a number of variations have been identified in SLC6A3, only one of these has been extensively studied as a potential predictor of individualized response to treatment with stimulants.

rs28363170 or 40-bp Variable-Number Tandem Repeat in the 3'UTR

rs28363170 (i.e., 40-bp variable-number tandem repeat [VNTR] in the 3'UTR) is the most well-studied variation of SLC6A3 and is located in exon 15. The two most common alleles of rs28363170 are the 9-repeat and the 10-repeat. However, eight other relatively rare alleles have been reported: 3-repeat, 5-repeat, 6-repeat, 7-repeat, 8-repeat, 11-repeat, 12-repeat, and 13 repeat (Sano et al., 1993).

GENOTYPIC VARIANCE ACROSS GEOGRAPHIC ANCESTRY

The allele frequency of rs28363170 (i.e., 40 bp VNTR in the 3' UTR) has been studied across many populations. The 10-repeat allele of rs28363170 is the most common variant in all populations, except for those living in some areas of the Middle East where the 9-repeat allele is the most common variant (Kang et al., 1999). In some South American samples, the 10-repeat allele is the only allele found.

The allele frequency of the 9-repeat allele of rs28363170 is the highest in Yemen, where it reaches 50%. In the Yemeni population, the relatively rare 3-repeat and 11-repeat alleles were both identified at a higher than anticipated frequency of about 3%. The allele frequency of the 10-repeat allele in Yemen was 44%.

In small isolated populations, such as the Mbuti in Africa, the allele frequency of the usually quite rare 7-repeat allele of rs28363170 has been documented to be as high as 33% (Kang et al., 1999). The very rare 13-repeat allele has only been reported in the remote Altai-Kizi population in Siberia (Mitchell et al., 2000).

ANTIDEPRESSANT MEDICATIONS

An association between rs28363170 (i.e., 40 bp VNTR in the 3' UTR) and response to the many antidepressant medications, including selective serotonin reuptake inhibitors, tricyclic antidepressants, venlafaxine, and mirtazapine has been reported (Kirchheiner et al., 2007). The highest response rate of 52% was reported for subjects who were homozygous for the 10-repeat allele of rs28363170. The response rate for subjects who were heterozygous for the 9-repeat allele and 10-repeat allele was 37%. The response rate for 9-repeat homozygous subjects was only 19%.

ANTIPSYCHOTIC MEDICATIONS

No consistent studies have linked variability in SLC6A3 with antipsychotic response or side effects.

STIMULANT MEDICATIONS

Methylphenidate

The 9-repeat and the 10-repeat alleles of rs28363170 (i.e., 40 bp VNTR in the 3' UTR) have been associated with differential responses to methylphenidate. An early report based on 16 children who responded to methylphenidate and 14 children who did not respond found that subjects who were homozygous for the 10-repeat allele were less likely to respond to methylphenidate than those with one or more copies of the 9-repeat allele (Winsberg & Comings, 1999). This finding was then replicated in a second small study (Roman et al., 2002). However, more recent studies of children with

ADHD have reported that the 10-repeat allele was associated with better response to methylphenidate in Irish children (Kirley et al., 2003) and in North American children of European origin (Stein et al., 2005). A better response in Canadian children with at least one 10-repeat allele has also been reported (Joober et al., 2007).

In the Netherlands, a small study of adult patients with ADHD who were treated with methylphenidate evaluated subjects with the 9-repeat, 10-repeat, and 11-repeat alleles (Kooij et al., 2008). The 10-repeat allele had an allele frequency of 70%, and 43% of the sample were homozygous for the 10-repeat allele. In contrast, only one subject was homozygous for the 9-repeat allele and no subjects were homozygous for the 11-repeat allele. Subjects who were heterozygous for the 9-repeat allele and 10-repeat allele (i.e., 9R/10R) were combined with subjects who were heterozygous for the 10-repeat allele and the 11-repeat allele (i.e., 10R/11R) into a single category. The overall response rate was low. Only 22% of subjects who were homozygous for the 10-repeat allele responded to methylphenidate, compared to 52% of all of the other subjects who were heterozygous (Kooij et al., 2008).

A study of Canadian adults explored variations of rs2836370 and its relationship to differential response of appetite suppression using methylphenidate. Some subjects who had one or two copies of the 9-repeat allele of rs28363170 reported effective appetite suppression. In contrast, no subjects who were homozygous for the 10-repeat allele reported appetite suppression (Davis et al., 2007).

Amphetamines

The effects of amphetamines in a North American sample of normal adult volunteers with diverse geographic ancestry has been studied in relation to variation in rs28363170. Subjects were administered placebo, 10 mg of dextroamphetamine, and 20 mg of dextroamphetamine. Subjects who were homozygous for the 9-repeat allele of rs28363170 (i.e., 40 bp VNTR in the 3' UTR) reported feeling less amphetamine "effect" when compared to subjects who were heterozygous for the 9-repeat and 10-repeat allele or those who were homozygous for the 10-repeat allele (Lott et al., 2005).

KEY CLINICAL CONSIDERATION

Although there has been interest in genotyping rs28363170 (i.e., 40 bp VNTR in the 3' UTR) to predict the response to methylphenidate, the results of multiple studies are difficult to interpret. However, it does appear that the 10-repeat allele may confer some greater risk for ADHD (Joober et al., 2007; Kirley et al., 2003; Stein et al., 2005), and patients who are homozygous for the 10-repeat allele may be more likely to respond to methylphenidate in some populations.

REFERENCES

Davis, C., Levitan, R. D., Kaplan, A. S., Carter, J., Reid, C., Curtis, C., et al. (2007). Dopamine transporter gene (DAT1) associated with appetite suppression to methylphenidate in a case–control study of binge eating disorder. *Neuropsychopharmacology, 32*, 2199–2206.

Greenwood, T. A., Alexander, M., Keck, P. E., McElroy, S., Sadovnick, A. D., Remick, R. A., et al. (2002). Segmental linkage disequilibrium within the dopamine transporter gene. *Molecular Psychiatry, 7*(2), 165–173.

Joober, R., Grizenko, N., Sengupta, S., Amor, L. B., Schmitz, N., Schwartz, G., et al. (2007). Dopamine transporter 3'-UTR VNTR genotype and ADHD: a pharmaco-behavioural genetic study with methylphenidate. *Neuropsychopharmacology, 32*(6), 1370–1376.

Kang, A. M., Palmatier, M. A., & Kidd, K. K. (1999). Global variation of a 40-bp VNTR in the 3'-untranslated region of the dopamine transporter gene (SLC6A3). *Biological Psychiatry, 46*(2), 151–160.

Kirchheiner, J., Nickchen, K., Sasse, J., Bauer, M., Roots, I., & Brockmoller, J. (2007). A 40-basepair VNTR polymorphism in the dopamine transporter (DAT1) gene and the rapid response to antidepressant treatment. *Pharmacogenomics Journal, 7*(1), 48–55.

Kirley, A., Lowe, N., Hawi, Z., Mullins, C., Daly, G., Waldman, I., et al. (2003). Association of the 480 bp DAT1 allele with methylphenidate response in a sample of Irish children with ADHD. *American Journal of Medical Genetics. Part B, Neuropsychiatric Genetics : The Official Publication of the International Society of Psychiatric Genetics, 121*(1), 50–54.

Kooij, J. S., Boonstra, A. M., Vermeulen, S. H., Heister, A. G., Burger, H., Buitelaar, J. K., & Franke, B. (2008). Response to methylphenidate in adults with ADHD is associated with a polymorphism in SLC6A3 (DAT1). *American Journal of Medical Genetics, Part B, Neuropsychiatric Genetics: The Official Publication of the International Society of Psychiatric Genetics, 147*(2), 201–208.

Lott, D. C., Kim, S.-J., Cook, E. H., Jr., & de Wit, H. (2005). Dopamine transporter gene associated with diminished subjective response to amphetamine. *Neuropsychopharmacology, 30*(3), 602–609.

Mitchell, R. J., Howlett, S., Earl, L., White, N. G., McComb, J., Schanfield, M. S., et al. (2000). Distribution of the 3' VNTR polymorphism in the human dopamine transporter gene in world populations. *Human Biology: An International Record of Research, 72*(2), 295–304.

Roman, T., Szobot, C., Martins, S., Biederman, J., Rohde, L., & Hutz, M. (2002). Dopamine transporter gene and response to methylphenidate in attention-deficit/hyperactivity disorder. *Pharmacogenetics, 12*(6), 497–499.

Sano, A., Kondoh, K., Kakimoto, Y., & Kondo, I. (1993). A 40-nucleotide repeat polymorphism in the human dopamine transporter gene. *Human Genetics, 91*(4), 405–406.

Stein, M. A., Waldman, I. D., Sarampote, C. S., Seymour, K. E., Robb, A. S., Conlon, C., et al. (2005). Dopamine transporter genotype and methylphenidate dose response in children with ADHD. *Neuropsychopharmacology, 30*(7), 1374–1382.

Winsberg, B. G., & Comings, D. E. (1999). Association of the dopamine transporter gene (DAT1) with poor methylphenidate response.[see comment]. *Journal of the American Academy of Child & Adolescent Psychiatry, 38*(12), 1474–1477.

11

THE SEROTONIN TRANSPORTER GENE

The serotonin transporter gene (SLC6A4) is frequently referred to as 5HTT or SERT. The SLC6A4 gene produces a protein that transfers serotonin from the synapse back into the neuron. Relatively high sequence homology exists between SLC6A4 and both SLC6A3 and SLC6A2 (Murphy, D.L. et al., 2004). The most widely studied genetic variation of SLC6A4 is an indel promoter polymorphism created by the deletion of 43 or 44 base pairs. This indel promoter polymorphism is frequently referred to in the literature as 5-HTTLPR or SERTPR. Variants of this indel promoter polymorphism are usually classified into two categories, which have been labeled the "long" allele or the "short" allele. The short allele is associated with reduced transcriptional efficiency, which results in decreased serotonin transporter expression (Lesch et al., 1996). In patients of European ancestry, it is now generally accepted that those who are homozygous for the long allele of the indel promoter polymorphism are more likely to respond to selective serotonin reuptake inhibitors (SSRIs) (Murphy, D.L. et al., 2004; Serretti et al., 2007).

LOCATION AND GENE VARIATION

SLC6A4 is located on chromosome 17. The specific location of the gene is on the long arm of chromosome 17 at 17q11.1-q12, which is very close to the centromere (Fig. 11.1).

SLC6A4 consists of approximately 37,800 nucleotides or 37.8 kilobases. It contains 15 exons, which are composed of 2,756 nucleotides. SLC6A4 codes for a polypeptide that is composed of 630 amino acids (Fig. 11.2).

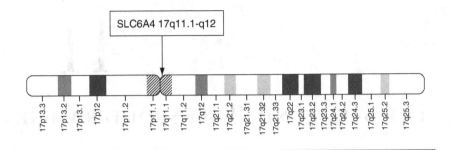

FIGURE 11.1. Chromosome 17 with arrow to designate the location of SLC6A4.

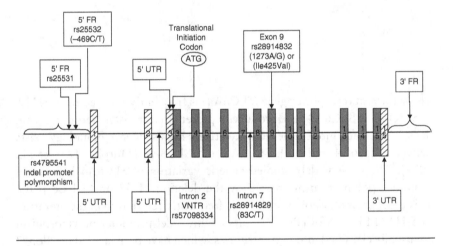

FIGURE 11.2. SLC6A4 structure illustrating the location of the 15 exons and the SNPs that define the most important SLC6A4 alleles.

Technical Discussion of SLC6A4 Variations

Each of the most well-studied SLC6A4 alleles is described in this technical discussion.

rs4795541 or indel promoter polymorphism or 5-HTTLPR or SERTPR or −2063 to −1714 44 bp deletion

rs4795541 (i.e., the indel promoter polymorphism) is often referred to as 5-HTTLPR or SERTPR. This variant is located in the promoter region of SLC6A4 and consists of a 43 or 44 bp deletion. Gene variants at this site are usually classified into two categories, which are referred to as the long alleles and the short alleles. The location of this polymorphism is between nucleotides −2063 and −1714.

The short alleles usually have 14 repeats of one of the characteristic sequences. The long alleles usually have 16 repeats. The indel promoter polymorphism is actually highly polymorphic. Fourteen allelic variants (14-A, 14-B, 14-C, 14-D, 15, 16-A, 16-B, 16-C, 16-D, 16-E, 16-F, 19, 20, and 22) have been identified in a cohort composed of both Japanese subjects and subjects of European ancestry (Nakamura et al., 2000).

rs25531

rs25531 is the result of an adenine to guanine change in the promoter region (Hu et al., 2007; Wendland et al., 2006). The guanine allele is associated with a decrease in promoter activity when it occurs in conjunction with the long allele of the indel promoter polymorphism.

rs25532 or −469C/T

rs25532 is the result of a cytosine to thymine change at nucleotide location −469 in the promoter region.

rs57098334 or 2nd Intron VNTR or STin2 VNTR

rs57098334 is a 17-bp variable-number tandem repeat (VNTR) which occurs in intron 2. While the 10- or 12-repeat sequences are the most common alleles, the 9- and 11- repeat sequences have also been reported.

rs28914829 or 83C/T

rs28914829 is a newly identified SNP which is the result of a cytosine to thymine change at nucleotide location 83 in intron 7. The allele frequency of the thymine allele was 2.5% in a sample of European ancestry. The thymine allele was found to be associated with a better response to citalopram in subjects who identified themselves as being "white" and "not Hispanic." However, this association may be due to linkage disequilibrium with the VNTR in the second intron (Mrazek et al., 2009).

rs28914832 or 1273A/G or Ile425Val

rs28914832 (i.e., Ile425Val) is located in the ninth exon and is the result of a change from an adenine to guanine at nucleotide location 1273. This nucleotide change results in an amino acid change from a isoleucine to a valine at amino acid position 425. The guanine allele has been associated with several neuropsychiatric phenotypes, including obsessive-compulsive disorder. The guanine allele has also been hypothesized to be associated with resistance to treatment with SSRIs (Delorme et al., 2005; Ozaki et al., 2003).

GENOTYPIC VARIANCE ACROSS GEOGRAPHIC ANCESTRY

The allele frequencies of the indel promoter polymorphism and the VNTR in the second intron have been studied in diverse ethnic and racial groups.

Indel Promoter Polymorphism

Considerable variability exists in the allele frequency of the long and short alleles of rs4795541 (i.e., the indel promoter polymorphism) in different populations

TABLE 11.1. Geographic variance in the allele frequency of the indel length variation of rs4795541

Geographic Ancestry	Long AlleleFrequency (%)	Short Allele Frequency (%)
African American	83	17
European American	60	40
Indian (Kolkata)	41	59
Afro-Caribbean (Tobago)	23	77
Han Chinese	26	74
Korean	23	77
Japanese	20	80

These allele frequencies are based on the mean calculation derived from reports in the literature. Approximately 15% of the long alleles in Japanese samples are classified as either "very long" or "extra long." Gelernter et al. (1997); Kunugi et al. (1997); Gelernter et al. (1999); Lotrich et al. (2003); Kim et al. (2006); Banerjee et al. (2006); and Li et al. (2007).

(Table 11.1). However, given the universality of both alleles, this variation must have occurred early in evolutionary history (Gelernter et al., 1999).

Considerable variability in allele frequencies of the long allele of rs4795541 has been reported in African American samples (Lotrich et al., 2003). For example, 77% of an African American sample from Western Pennsylvania had the long allele, as compared to 87% of an African American sample from South Carolina.

2nd Intron 17 bp VNTR

Although the two most common alleles of the 17 bp VNTR of the second intron (i.e., 10-repeat and 12-repeat) are found in all cultures, the less common 9-repeat allele is found only in individuals of European or African ancestry (Gelernter et al., 1999) (Table 11.2). The even rarer 11-repeat allele has only been identified in individuals with Sub-Saharan ancestry.

TABLE 11.2. Variability in allele frequencies of the 2nd intron VNTR in six geographical populations

Geographic Ancestry	9-repeat Frequency (%)	10-repeat Frequency (%)	12-repeat Frequency (%)
European American	1	47	52
Indian; mixed castes (Kolkata)	<0.1	29	71
African American	1	26	73
Korean	<0.1	10	90
Han Chinese	<0.1	8	92
Japanese	<0.1	2	98

These allele frequencies are based on the mean calculation derived from reports in the literature. Gelernter et al. (1997); Kunugi et al. (1997); Gelernter et al. (1999); Kim et al. (2005); Banerjee et al. (2006); and Li et al. (2007).

ANTIDEPRESSANT MEDICATIONS

rs4795541 variation has been repeatedly associated with SSRI response in samples of European ancestry. This genetic variation also predicts responses to other antidepressant medications that influence availability of serotonin.

Nortriptyline

A Korean study examined the association between response to the tricyclic antidepressant nortriptyline and rs4795541. The response rate of subjects who were homozygous for the short form of the indel promoter polymorphism was 76%, as compared to the 48% response rate of patients who were heterozygous for the long and short polymorphism. The response rate of patients who were homozygous for the long polymorphism was 30%. Those subjects who were homozygous for the short form of the indel polymorphism in SLC6A4 and also homozygous for the guanine allele of rs5569 (i.e., 1287G/A) in SLC6A2 had a response rate of 89%. The worst response rate for patients treated with nortriptyline was 22%, which occurred in subjects who had one or more of the long alleles of the indel promoter polymorphism in SLC6A4 and had one or more copies of the adenine allele of rs5569 (i.e., 1287G/A) in SLC6A2 (Kim et al., 2006).

Citalopram and Escitalopram

Citalopram is a serotonin reuptake inhibitor that is widely used in clinical practice and consists of a racemic mixture of the l-isomer and the d-isomer. Escitalopram is a serotonin reuptake inhibitor that contains only the active l-isomer of citalopram.

The response of a large cohort of patients with major depression who were treated with citalopram using a standard protocol has been analyzed. Patients who defined their ancestry as being "white" and "not Hispanic" were more likely to respond to citalopram if they were homozygous for the long allele of rs4795541 (i.e., the indel promoter polymorphism) (Mrazek et al., 2009). This group also was more likely to respond to citalopram if they had a copy of the 9-repeat allele of the 17 bp VNTR in the second intron in combination with the 12-repeat allele. About 76% of individuals who were homozygous for the long allele of the indel promoter polymorphism and who had the *9/*12 genotype for the second intron VNTR experienced a complete remission of their depression when treated with citalopram.

A different analysis of this data set that pooled white Hispanics with white non-Hispanics did not demonstrate a statistically significant association between remission and having the homozygous long allele genotype (Kraft et al., 2007). This alternative analysis also used a less rigorous definition of remission, as it included subjects who had an early remission of symptoms, but subsequently relapsed within the first 8 weeks of treatment.

In a small Spanish sample of patients with major depressive disorder, no association between the indel promoter variant and response to treatment with escitalopram was demonstrated. However, patients in this cohort who had the short/short indel polymorphism genotype and were homozygous for the guanine allele of rs6295 (i.e., –1019C/G) in HTR1A did respond less well than did those who were homozygous for the long allele of the indel promoter polymorphism genotype in SLC6A4 and who were homozygous for the cytosine allele of rs6295 in HTR1A (Arias et al., 2005).

Sertraline and Fluoxetine

Paradoxically, in a Korean sample of patients with depression, patients with the short/short indel promoter polymorphism genotype in SLC6A4 responded more positively to treatment with sertraline and fluoxetine when compared to subjects with the long allele (Kim et al., 2006). This association is quite different from the consistently documented association of better response in patients of European ancestry with the long allele (Serretti et al., 2007). Although there is no widely accepted explanation for this difference, some variability exists in the classification of the alleles in the Korean study. In the Korean study, the short category was restricted to those individuals who were homogenous for alleles composed of 14-repeats. In contrast, subjects with 16-repeats, 18-repeats, 20-repeats, and 22-repeats were all classified as having the "long allele." In this Korean sample, the effect of variation in the second intron VNTR of SLC6A4 was also assessed. Again, the subjects were dichotomized into those with the short alleles and those with the long alleles. Subjects with either the 9-repeat or 10-repeat allele were classified as having short alleles. In contrast, subjects with 12-repeat alleles were classified as having the long alleles. Patients who were homozygous for the long 12-repeat allele had a response rate of 69%, compared to a response rate of only 9% for subjects who did not have this genotype.

Fluvoxamine

In an early pharmacogenomic study of Italian inpatients with depression that included patients with psychotic symptoms, those patients who were homozygous for the short allele of the indel promoter polymorphism of SLC6A4 responded less well to treatment with fluvoxamine than did patients who were heterozygous for the long allele and short allele or those who were homozygous for the long allele (Smeraldi et al., 1998). All patients, including those who were homozygous for the short allele, responded more favorably if they were additionally treated with pindolol, which is a serotonin autoreceptor agonist.

In a second replication study of Italian patients with a range of severity of depressive symptoms, patients who were homozygous for the short allele of the indel promoter polymorphism of SLC6A4 responded less well to treatment with fluvoxamine (Zanardi et al., 2001). Patients who were homozygous for the short allele of the indel polymorphism genotype again responded more positively to fluvoxamine if they concurrently received an augmenting dose of pindolol.

Lithium Augmentation

A German study of the treatment of depressed adults reported that those who were homozygous for the short allele of the indel promoter polymorphism of SLC6A4 did not respond as well to antidepressants (Stamm et al., 2008). Patients who were heterozygous for the long and short allele of the indel promoter polymorphism, as well as patients who were homozygous for the long allele, responded better to antidepressants. However, patients who were homozygous for the short allele showed a particularly good response to lithium augmentation.

Meta-analysis of Selective Serotonin Reuptake Inhibitor Studies

A review of 15 studies examining the implications of variations in the indel promoter polymorphism of SLC6A4 concluded that patients of European ancestry who were homozygous for the short indel allele consistently responded less well to treatment with SSRIs than did patients who were homozygous for the long allele of the indel promoter polymorphism (Serretti et al., 2007). Patients with one long copy and one short copy of the indel promoter polymorphism often, but not always, had an intermediate response. A study designed to examine the specific pattern of symptom improvement suggested that patients who were homozygous for the short allele of the indel promoter polymorphism were less likely to show improvement in core symptoms of depression and somatic anxiety symptoms (Serretti et al., 2007). Further classification of rare variants that are routinely classified simply as being "long" may further increase the predictive ability of genotyping the indel promoter polymorphism of SLC6A4 (Smeraldi et al., 2006).

ADVERSE EFFECTS OF ANTIDEPRESSANT MEDICATION

Depressed patients treated with citalopram have also been examined to determine whether a relationship between the indel promoter genotype and development of gastrointestinal side effects, including diarrhea, could be demonstrated. Subjects who identified themselves as white and who had at least one copy of the long allele of the indel promoter genotype were divided into two separate groups based on the rs25531 genotype. In an earlier paper, this group had reported that the guanine allele of rs25531 created a functional AP2 transcription factor–binding site that effectively decreased the expression of the long allele to be at an equivalent level as the short allele (Hu et al., 2006). In their later publication, they reported that white subjects who were homozygous for the long allele of SLC6A4 and who also had one or more copies of the adenine allele of rs25531 were less likely to report gastrointestinal side effects (Hu et al., 2007).

A small German study of psychiatric inpatients with the diagnosis of depression reported associations between side effects and the two most commonly studied genetic variants of SLC6A4 (Popp et al., 2006). Those patients who were treated with antidepressants that block the serotonin transporter had more side effects if they had one or more copies of the short allele of the indel promoter polymorphism when compared to patients who were homozygous for the long allele. Those patients who were homozygous for the 10-repeat VNTR in the second intron of SLC6A4 had more side effects when compared to other VNTR genotypes. A "high-risk" group was defined as being both homozygous for the short indel genotype and homozygous for the 10-repeat allele of the VNTR variant. Evaluating the response to antidepressant medication in this risk group revealed that 63% reported having side effects. A contrasting low-risk group was defined as being homozygous for the long indel allele and having one or more copies of the 12-repeat allele. None of the subjects in the low risk group experienced side effects.

In a study of depressed geriatric patients who were treated with paroxetine, an association between being homozygous for the short allele of the indel promoter polymorphism of SLC6A4 and having more side effects was reported (Murphy, G.M. et al., 2004). Patients who were homozygous for the short allele were more likely to discontinue participation in the study based on having more severe side effects, which included gastrointestinal symptoms, fatigue, agitation, sweating, and dizziness.

Genetic variation of the indel promoter polymorphism of SLC6A4 was associated with a lifetime history of antidepressant-induced mania in a population of 305 patients with bipolar affective disorder (Rousseva et al., 2003). A statistical association was not demonstrated to exist between the short allele of the indel polymorphism and antidepressant-induced mania. However, the short allele did occur more frequently in patients with antidepressant-induced mania. Additionally, an association existed between the short allele of the indel polymorphism and lifetime history of rapid cycling in a subsample of patients.

A more recent study of Spanish patients with depression reported that antidepressant-induced mania occurred more frequently in subjects who were homozygous for the short allele of the indel promoter polymorphism when compared to other rs4795541 genotypes (Masoliver et al., 2006). Of the 37 identified subjects with antidepressant-induced mania, 19 subjects had been treated with tricyclic antidepressants, nine had been treated with selective serotonin reuptake inhibitors, five with monoamine oxidase inhibitors, and four subjects had been treated with venlafaxine.

A relationship between being homozygous for the short allele of the indel promoter polymorphism of SLC6A4 and suicidal symptoms has been reported. However, the hypothesis that this association was the result of the use of antidepressant medications has not been demonstrated.

ANTIPSYCHOTIC MEDICATION

Clozapine

rs4795541 (i.e., the indel promoter variant) of SLC6A4 has been reported to be associated with clozapine response when this genotype was included in a panel of six gene variants. The analysis of these six variants resulted in a 77% successful prediction of clozapine response (Arranz et al., 2000).

STIMULANT MEDICATION

Methylphenidate

Methylphenidate, a stimulant used to treat attention-deficit hyperactivity disorder (ADHD), has a primary action of blocking the reuptake of dopamine. This results in an increase in synaptic dopamine, which antagonizes the release of prolactin. In contrast to dopamine, serotonin is an agonist that increases the release of prolactin. In a German study, 47 children who were hospitalized for ADHD were genotyped for both the indel promoter polymorphism of SLC6A4 and the 48 bp VNTR of dopamine D4 receptor gene (DRD4) while being treated with methylphenidate (Seeger et al., 2001). Subjects who were homozygous for the long indel allele of SLC6A4 and had one or two copies of the 7-repeat allele of the DRD4 VNTR were less likely to respond to methylphenidate when compared to children with other genotypes. The best response to methylphenidate occurred in children who were homozygous for the short allele of the indel promoter polymorphism who also had one or more copies of the 7-repeat allele of DRD4 VNTR.

Clinical Implications

Patients of European ancestry who are homozygous for the long allele of the indel promoter polymorphism are more likely to respond to antidepressant medications that act by inhibiting the reuptake of serotonin, when compared to patients who are homozygous for the short indel alleles. Some evidence exists to support the conclusion that these patients are even more likely to respond if they are also homozygous for the adenine allele of rs25531.

Clinical Case 9

A 36-year-old woman experienced an acute onset of depressive symptoms. Her Beck Depression Inventory-II score of 24 suggested that her depression was moderately severe. However, she was not suicidal. She was born in Boston, but both of her parents had immigrated to the United States from Italy. She had never been previously treated for depressive illness, but her mother and older sister had both experienced episodes of depression. Her mother had responded well to fluoxetine and her older sister had responded well to citalopram. Pharmacogenomic testing was ordered prior to selection of an antidepressant medication (Table 11.3).

This patient has all three SLC6A4 genotypes associated with better response to antidepressants. Specifically, she was homozygous for the long

---

TABLE 11.3. Pharmacogenomic report of case 9

Pharmacogenomic Report of Case 9			
Gene	Gene Variant	Genotype	Clinical Implication
CYP2D6	N/A	*1/*2A	Extensive CYP2D6 metabolizer
CYP2C19	N/A	*1/*17	Extensive CYP2C19 metabolizer
CYP2C9	N/A	*2/*2	Poor CYP2C9 metabolizer
CYP1A2	N/A	*1A/*1A	Extensive CYP1A2 metabolizer
COMT	rs4680	G/G	High activity
SLC6A2	rs5569	G/G	Better antidepressant response
SLC6A4	rs4795541	Long/Long	Higher activity
SLC6A4	2nd intron VNTR	12-repeat/ 12-repeat	Better antidepressant response
SLC6A4	rs25531	A/A	Better antidepressant response

allele of the indel promoter variant, homozygous for the 12-repeat allele of the 2nd intron VNTR, and homozygous for the adenine allele of rs25531. Her CYP2D6 and CYP2C19 genotypes also suggested that she could metabolize citalopram with no difficulty. Based on her genotype, it is highly likely that she would respond well to either citalopram or escitalopram, and that she could tolerate treatment with these medications at standard or even relatively high doses.

Clinical Case 10

A 41-year-old Korean married woman presented for treatment of a rather sudden onset of acute depression. She had experienced a previous untreated episode of depression following the birth of her first child, which resolved within 3 months. Although she felt despondent and reported an inability to sleep through the night, she denied any suicidal ideation. Her physician was familiar with the work of Dr. Kim at Samsung Medical Center, and he consequently ordered a pharmacogenomic profile (Table 11.4) before selecting an antidepressant (Kim et al., 2006).

Based on studies of Korean subjects, this patient has an increased probability of having a positive response to treatment with nortriptyline. She would also be expected to have a positive response to an SSRI (Kim et al., 2006), but she is unlikely to tolerate either CYP2D6 or CYP2C19 substrate medications at standard doses. However, given that she is an extensive metabolizer of CYP1A2 substrates, treatment with fluvoxamine at a standard dose would be a safe choice.

TABLE 11.4. Pharmacogenomic report of case 10

Pharmacogenomic Report of Case 10			
Gene	Gene Variant	Genotype	Clinical Implication
CYP2D6	N/A	*4/*4	Poor CYP2D6 metabolizer
CYP2C19	N/A	*3/*8	Poor CYP2C19 metabolizer
CYP2C9	N/A	*1/*2	Intermediate CYP2C9 metabolizer
CYP1A2	N/A	*1A/*1A	Extensive CYP1A2 metabolizer
COMT	rs4680	A/A	Low activity
SLC6A2	rs5569	A/A	Worse antidepressant response
SLC6A4	rs4795541	Short/Short	Low activity
SLC6A4	2nd intron VNTR	10-repeat/ 10-repeat	Worse antidepressant response
SLC6A4	rs25531	G/G	Worse antidepressant response

KEY CLINICAL CONSIDERATIONS

- In patients of European ancestry, those who are homozygous for the long allele of the indel promoter polymorphism of rs4795541 are more likely to respond to SSRIs than are patients who are homozygous for the short allele.
- Variations of the VNTR of the second intron of SLC6A4, such as having the 9-repeat/12-repeat genotype, may also improve the probability of response to citalopram and escitalopram.

REFERENCES

Arias, B., Catalan, R., Gasto, C., Gutierrez, B., & Fananas, L. (2005). Evidence for a combined genetic effect of the 5-HT1A receptor and serotonin transporter genes in the clinical outcome of major depressive patients treated with citalopram. *Journal of Psychopharmacology, 19*(2), 166–172.

Arranz, M. J., Munro, J., Birkett, J., Bolonna, A., Mancama, D. T., Sodhi, M., et al. (2000). Pharmacogenetic prediction of clozapine response. *Lancet, 355,* 1615–1616.

Banerjee, E., Sinha, S., Chatterjee, A., Gangopadhyay, P. K., Singh, M., & Nandagopal, K. (2006). A family-based study of Indian subjects from Kolkata reveals allelic association of the serotonin transporter intron-2 (STin2) polymorphism and attention-deficit-hyperactivity disorder (ADHD). *American Journal of Medical Genetics. Part B, Neuropsychiatric Genetics, 141B*(4), 361–366.

Delorme, R., Betancur, C., Wagner, M., Krebs, M. O., Gorwood, P., Pearl, P., et al. (2005). Support for the association between the rare functional variant I425V of the serotonin transporter gene and susceptibility to obsessive compulsive disorder. *Molecular Psychiatry, 10*(12), 1059–1061.

Gelernter, J., Cubells, J. F., Kidd, J. R., Pakstis, A. J., & Kidd, K. K. (1999). Population studies of polymorphisms of the serotonin transporter protein gene. *American Journal of Medical Genetics, 88*(1), 61–66.

Gelernter, J., Kranzler, H., & Cubells, J. F. (1997). Serotonin transporter protein (SLC6A4) allele and haplotype frequencies and linkage disequilibria in African- and European-American and Japanese populations and in alcohol-dependent subjects. *Human Genetics, 101*(2), 243–246.

Hu, X. Z., Lipsky, R. H., Zhu, G., Akhtar, L. A., Taubman, J., Greenberg, B. D., et al. (2006). Serotonin transporter promoter gain-of-function genotypes are linked to obsessive-compulsive disorder. *American Journal of Human Genetics, 78*(5), 815–826.

Hu, X. Z., Rush, A. J., Charney, D., Wilson, A. F., Sorant, A. J., Papanicolaou, G. J., et al. (2007). Association between a functional serotonin transporter promoter polymorphism and citalopram treatment in adult outpatients with major depression. *Archives of General Psychiatry, 64*(7), 783–792.

Kim, S. J., Badner, J., Cheon, K. A., Kim, B. N., Yoo, H. J., Kim, S. J., et al. (2005). Family-based association study of the serotonin transporter gene polymorphisms in Korean ADHD trios. *American Journal of Medical Genetics Part B, Neuropsychiatric Genetics: The Official Publication of the International Society of Psychiatric Genetics, 139*(1), 14–18.

Kim, H., Lim, S. W., Kim, S., Kim, J. W., Chang, Y. H., Carroll, B. J., & Kim, D. K. (2006). Monoamine transporter gene polymorphisms and antidepressant response in Koreans with late-life depression. *JAMA: The Journal of the American Medical Association, 296*(13), 1609–1618.

Kraft, J. B., Peters, E. J., Slager, S. L., Jenkins, G. D., Reinalda, M. S., McGrath, P. J., & Hamilton, S. P. (2007). Analysis of association between the serotonin transporter and antidepressant response in a large clinical sample. *Biological Psychiatry, 61*(6), 734–742.

Kunugi, H., Hattori, M., Kato, T., Tatsumi, M., Sakai, T., Sasaki, T., et al. (1997). Serotonin transporter gene polymorphisms: ethnic difference and possible association with bipolar affective disorder. *Molecular Psychiatry, 2*(6), 457–462.

Li, J., Wang, Y., Zhou, R., Zhang, H., Yang, L., Wang, B., & Faraone, S. V. (2007). Association between polymorphisms in serotonin transporter gene and attention deficit hyperactivity disorder in Chinese Han subjects. *American Journal of Medical Genetics Part B, Neuropsychiatric Genetics: The Official Publication of the International Society of Psychiatric Genetics, 144*(1), 14–19.

Lesch, K. P., Bengel, D., Heils, A., Sabol, S. Z., Greenberg, B. D., Petri, S., et al. (1996). Association of anxiety-related traits with a polymorphism in the serotonin transporter gene regulatory region. *Science, 274*(5292), 1527–1531.

Lotrich, F., Pollock, B., & Ferrell, R. (2003). Serotonin transporter promoter polymorphism in African Americans: allele frequencies and implications for treatment. *American Journal of Pharmacogenomics, 3*(2), 145–147.

Masoliver, E., Menoyo, A., Perez, V., Volpini, V., Rio, E. D., Perez, J., Alvarez, E., & Baiget, M. (2006). Serotonin transporter linked promoter (polymorphism) in the serotonin transporter gene may be associated with antidepressant-induced mania in bipolar disorder. *Psychiatric Genetics, 16*(1), 25–29.

Mrazek, D. A., Rush, A. J., Biernacka, J. M., O'Kane, D. J., Cunningham, J. M., Wieben, E. D., et al. (2009). SLC6A4 variation and citalopram response. *American Journal of Medical Genetics. Part B, Neuropsychiatric Genetics: The Official Publication of the International Society of Psychiatric Genetics, 150*, 341–351.

Murphy, D. L., Lerner, A., Rudnick, G., & Lesch, K. P. (2004). Serotonin transporter: gene, genetic disorders, and pharmacogenetics. *Molecular interventions, 4*(2), 109–123.

Murphy, G. M., Hollander, S. B., Rodrigues, H. E., Kremer, C., & Schatzberg, A. F. (2004). Effects of the serotonin transporter gene promoter polymorphism on mirtazapine and paroxetine efficacy and adverse events in geriatric major depression. *Archives of General Psychiatry, 61*, 1163–1169.

Nakamura, M., Ueno, S., Sano, A., & Tanabe, H. (2000). The human serotonin transporter gene linked polymorphism (5-HTTLPR) shows ten novel allelic variants. *Molecular Psychiatry, 5*(1), 32–38.

Ozaki, N., Goldman, D., Kaye, W. H., Plotnicov, K., Greenberg, B. D., Lappalainen, J., & Rudnick, G. (2003). Serotonin transporter missense mutation associated with a complex neuropsychiatric phenotype. *Molecular Psychiatry, 8*(11), 933–936.

Popp, J., Leucht, S., Heres, S., & Steimer, W. (2006). Serotonin transporter polymorphisms and side effects in antidepressant therapy—a pilot study. *Pharmacogenomics, 7*(2), 159–166.

Rousseva, A., Henry, C., van den Bulke, D., Fournier, G., Laplanche, J. L., Leboyer, M., et al. (2003). Antidepressant-induced mania, rapid cycling and the serotonin transporter gene polymorphism. *The Pharmacogenomics Journal, 3*(2), 101–104.

Seeger, G., Schloss, P., & Schmidt, M. H. (2001). Marker gene polymorphisms in hyperkinetic disorder—predictors of clinical response to treatment with methylphenidate? *Neuroscience letters 313*(1–2), 45–48.

Serretti, A., Kato, M., De Ronchi, D., & Kinoshita, T. (2007). Meta-analysis of serotonin transporter gene promoter polymorphism (5-HTTLPR) association with selective serotonin reuptake inhibitor efficacy in depressed patients. *Molecular Psychiatry, 12*(3), 247–257.

Smeraldi, E., Serretti, A., Artioli, P., Lorenzi, C., & Catalano, M. (2006). Serotonin transporter gene-linked polymorphic region: possible pharmacogenetic implications of rare variants. *Psychiatric Genetics, 16*(4), 153–158.

Smeraldi, E., Zanardi, R., Benedetti, F., Bella, D., Perez, J., & Catalano, M. (1998). Polymorphism within the promoter of the serotonin transporter gene and antidepressant efficacy of fluvoxamine. *Molecular psychiatry, 3*, 508–511.

Stamm, T. J., Adli, M., Kirchheiner, J., Smolka, M. N., Kaiser, R., Tremblay, P. B., & Bauer, M. (2008). Serotonin transporter gene and response to lithium augmentation in depression. *Psychiatric Genetics, 18*(2), 92–97.

Wendland, J., Martin, B., Kruse, M., Lesch, K.-P., & Murphy, D. (2006). Simultaneous genotyping of four functional loci of human SLC6A4, with a reappraisal of 5-HTTLPR and rs25531. *Molecular Psychiatry, 11*(3), 224–226.

Zanardi, R., Serretti, A., Rossini, D., Franchini, L., Cusin, C., Lattuada, E., Dotoli, D., & Smeraldi, E. (2001). Factors affecting fluvoxamine antidepressant activity: influence of pindolol and 5-HTTLPR in delusional and nondelusional depression. *Biological Psychiatry, 50*(5), 323–330.

V

THE SEROTONIN RECEPTOR GENES

12

THE SEROTONIN 1A
RECEPTOR GENE

Variations in the serotonin 1A receptor gene (HTR1A) have been associated with mood disorder, suicidal behavior, and antidepressant response. The distribution of HTR1A receptors in the brain is consistent with our understanding that these receptors play a role in both cognition and emotional regulation. HTR1A receptors are present in high density in the dorsal and median raphe nuclei, the cortex, the hypothalamus, and the amygdala (Hensler, 2003).

LOCATION AND GENE VARIATION

The HTR1A gene is located on chromosome 5. The specific location of the gene is on the long arm of chromosome 5 at 5q11.2–q13 (Fig. 12.1).

The HTR1A gene consists of 1,269 nucleotides or approximately 1.27 kilobases. It contains only one exon. HTR1A codes for a polypeptide composed of 422 amino acids (Fig. 12.2). HTR1A is a very small gene and with only one exon, it is the simplest gene reviewed in this book.

Table 12.1 provides a list of the most well-studied HTR1A alleles and includes both ancestral and mutant alleles. See the technical discussion for a description of each allele.

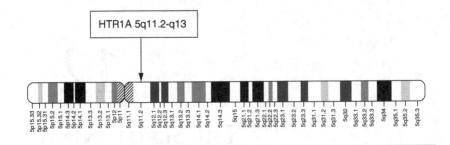

FIGURE 12.1. Chromosome 5 with arrow to designate the location of the HTR1A gene.

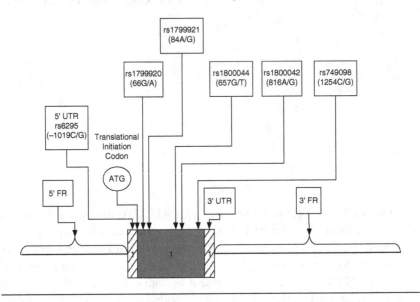

FIGURE 12.2. HTR1A structure illustrating the location of the one exon and the single nucleotide polymorphisms that define the most important HTR1A alleles.

TABLE 12.1. The locations of nucleotide changes that define the most well-studied HTR1A alleles

refSNP ID & Aliases	Nucleotide Location	Ancestral Allele	Mutant Variant
rs6295 or −1019C/G	−1019	C	G
rs1799920 or 66G/A or Gly22Ser	66	G	A
rs1799921 or 84A/G or Ile28Val	84	A	G
rs1800044 or 657G/T or Arg219Leu	657	G	T
rs1800042 or 816A/G or Gly272Asp	816	A	G
rs749098 or 1254C/G or Asn417Lys	1254	C	G

Technical Discussion of HTR1A Variations

Each of the most well-studied HTR1A alleles is described in this technical discussion.

rs6295 or –1019C/G (Previously Reported As –1018C/G)

rs6295 is the most widely studied HTR1A variant. rs6295 is the result of a cytosine to guanine change in the promoter region at nucleotide position –1019. Although differential expression between the cytosine allele and the guanine allele has been reported, the degree of differential expression has not been definitively established (Lesch & Gutnecht, 2004).

rs1799920 or 66G/A or Gly22Ser

rs1799920 is the result of a guanine to adenine change at nucleotide location 66 in exon 1. This change results in a change from a glycine to a serine at amino acid position 22.

rs1799921 or 84A/G or Ile28Val

rs179921 is the result of an adenine to guanine change at nucleotide location 84 in exon 1. This change results in the coding of a valine rather than an isoleucine at amino acid position 28.

rs1800044 or 657G/T or Arg219Leu

rs1800044 is the result of a guanine to thymine change at nucleotide position 657 in exon 1. This results in an amino acid change of a leucine to an arginine at amino acid position 219, which is located in the third intracellular loop of the HTR1A receptor. The third intracellular loop is the location believed to be the site of G protein-coupling on the receptor and consequently is thought to have a major effect on receptor-mediated signal transduction. rs1800044 was initially identified in a patient with Tourette syndrome (Lam et al., 1996).

rs1800042 or 816A/G or Gly272Asp

rs1800042 is the result of an adenine to guanine change at nucleotide location 816 in exon 1. This change results in an amino acid change from a glycine to an aspartic acid at amino acid position 272. Although this variant was documented to be quite rare in a Chinese sample, rs1800042 is in strong linkage disequilibrium with the more extensively studied rs6295 (i.e., –1019C/G).

rs749098 or 1254C/G or Asn417Lys

rs749098 is the result of a cytosine to guanine change at nucleotide location 1254 in exon 1. This change results in an amino acid change from an asparagine to a lysine at amino acid position 417 (Lam et al., 1996).

GENOTYPIC VARIANCE ACROSS GEOGRAPHIC ANCESTRY

The guanine and cytosine alleles of rs6295 (i.e., –1019C/G) have been reported in an Italian population to be quite evenly distributed, with 51% of the population having the guanine allele and 49% having the cytosine allele (Serretti et al., 2004). A similar allelic distribution was reported in a Canadian sample (Lemonde et al., 2004).

A report of the analysis of a Chinese sample of depressed patients revealed more subjects with the guanine allele of rs6295 (Yu et al., 2006). In this sample, the mean allele frequency of the guanine allele was 78%, as compared to an allele frequency of 22% for the cytosine allele. In this same Chinese sample, the allele frequency of rs1800042 (i.e., Gly272Asp) was also assessed and an allele frequency of the adenine allele was reported to be 99% with only 1% of the sample having the guanine allele.

Allelic variability of HTR1A has been assessed in an African American sample (Glatt et al., 2004). This data supports the conclusion that considerable variability exists in different African populations.

ANTIDEPRESSANT MEDICATIONS

Patients who are homozygous for the cytosine allele of rs6295 (i.e., –1019C/G) have been reported to have a better response to antidepressant medication than patients with one or more copies of the guanine allele.

Fluvoxamine

A positive antidepressant response to fluvoxamine has been linked to being homozygous for the cytosine allele of rs6295 (i.e., –1019C/G) in patients with bipolar disorder (Serretti et al., 2004).

Citalopram

A positive association has been reported in the interaction of HTR1A and SLC6A4 in patients with major depression treated with citalopram. As predicted from independent studies of these two genes, patients with the active indel promoter long variant of SLC6A4 and the cytosine allele of rs6295 did better than patients who were homozygous for the less active indel promoter short allele of SLC6A4 and who were homozygous for the guanine allele of rs6295 (Arias et al., 2005). Patients who were homozygous for both the short allele of SLC6A4 and the guanine allele of rs6295 had a remission rate of only 17%, suggesting that these patients should be treated with an alternative antidepressant medication.

Fluoxetine

A more positive response to treatment with fluoxetine was reported in a Chinese sample of patients with depression (Yu et al., 2006). Subjects who were homozygous for the cytosine allele of rs6295 were most likely to respond to fluoxetine. A relationship was also noted between having the adenine allele of rs1800042 (i.e., Gly272Asp) and a positive response to treatment with fluoxetine.

Buspirone

Buspirone is a HTR1A receptor agonist available in the United States for the treatment of depression and anxiety. Patients with the thymine allele (i.e., the leucine allele) of rs1800044 (i.e., Arg219Leu) responded less well to buspirone than those with the guanine allele (i.e., the arginine allele) (Brüss et al., 2005).

Flibanserin

Flibanserin is an HTR1A agonist that is also an HTR2A antagonist. Although flibanserin is used as an antidepressant medication in Europe, it has not been approved for use in the United States (Invernizzi et al., 2003). Depressed subjects with one or two copies of the cytosine allele of rs6295 responded more favorably to flibanserin than did subjects who were homozygous for the guanine allele (Lemonde et al., 2004).

ANTIPSYCHOTIC MEDICATIONS

Many antipsychotic medications do not have a strong affinity to the HTR1A receptor. However, ziprasidone (Duncan et al., 1999) and aripiprazole (Jordan et al., 2002; Stark et al., 2007) do have strong affinities (Table 12.2). The limited pharmacogenomic data that have been reported support the hypothesis that the cytosine allele of rs6295 (i.e., –1019C/G) is associated with a better response to antipsychotic medication.

Risperidone and Olanzapine

Schizophrenic subjects who are homozygous for the cytosine allele of rs6295 responded to risperidone and olanzapine with a greater improvement of

TABLE 12.2. Antipsychotic drug affinity (ability to bind to receptor) in nM

Antipsychotic Drugs	Affinity
Aripiprazole	High (4.2)
Ziprasidone	High (2.5)
Clozapine	Low (140)
Risperidone	Low (210)
Quetiapine	Low (230)
Olanzapine	Low (2100)
Haloperidol	Low (3600)

negative symptoms than those with a copy of the guanine allele (Reynolds et al., 2006). However, this rs6295 genotype did not predict improvement of positive symptoms. Subjects in this study also were reported to have greater improvement in collateral depressive symptoms if they were homozygous for the cytosine allele of rs6295.

CLINICAL IMPLICATIONS

Currently, the primary use of the genotyping of HTR1A is to clarify the probability of benefit for specific psychotropic medications. For example, patients who are poor metabolizers of both 2D6 substrate and 2C19 substrate antidepressant medications provide a considerable challenge for treating depression. Information about pharmacodynamic probability of response can be used to help identify an antidepressant that has a higher probability of resulting in remission. Fluvoxamine and mirtazapine are two antidepressant medications that are primarily metabolized by other enzymes. Making the selection between these two antidepressant medications can be facilitated by the identification of specific variants in HTR1A.

Clinical Case 11

A 27-year-old male patient of Norwegian ancestry developed severe depression after he lost his position as an investment banker. He had previously been prescribed fluoxetine, and had experienced nausea and sexual side effects. He subsequently was treated with venlafaxine but discontinued taking his medication when his dose was increased to 150 mg and he developed severe headaches. Pharmacogenomic testing was ordered (Table 12.3).

TABLE 12.3. Pharmacogenomic report of case 11

Pharmacogenomic Report of Case 11			
Gene	Gene Variant	Genotype	Clinical Implication
CYP2D6	N/A	*4/*6	Poor CYP2D6 metabolizer
CYP2C19	N/A	*2/*8	Poor CYP2C19 metabolizer
CYP2C9	N/A	*1/*1	Intermediate CYP2C9 metabolizer
CYP1A2	N/A	*1F/*1F	Extensive CYP1A2 metabolizer
COMT	rs4680	A/A	Low Activity
SLC6A2	rs5569	G/G	Better antidepressant response
SLC6A4	Indel promoter	Long/Long	Better antidepressant response
SLC6A4	rs4795541	9-repeat/9-repeat	Better antidepressant response
SLC6A4	rs25531	A/A	Better antidepressant response
HTR1A	rs6295	C/C	Better antidepressant response

The pharmacogenomic results support the use of fluvoxamine in this patient, as fluvoxamine is a CYP1A2 substrate medication. In addition, this patient is homozygous both for alleles of SLC6A4 that increase gene expression and for the cytosine allele of rs6295 in HTR1A. These genotypes specifically predicts a good response to fluvoxamine in patients of European ancestry. The medication could be metabolized by this patient despite his 2D6 and 2C19 genotypes.

Mirtazapine would also be a reasonable choice of an antidepressant, as his pharmacogenomic report suggests that he could metabolize this medication as well. However, no studies of target genes suggest that this patient would have a superior response with mirtazapine.

Another treatment strategy would be to consider using citalopram. While the patient is a poor CYP2C19 metabolizer, and citalopram is metabolized predominantly by the CYP2C19 enzyme, evidence demonstrates that patients who are poor metabolizers and are willing to tolerate a standard dose of citalopram, despite their side effects, have a quite high probability of achieving remission of their depressive symptoms (Mrazek et al., 2008).

KEY CLINICAL CONSIDERATION

Patients who are homozygous for the cytosine allele of rs6295 (i.e., –1019C/G) are more likely to respond to treatment with both a selective serotonin reuptake inhibitor (SSRI) and a serotonin 1A receptor agonist than are patients who are homozygous for the guanine allele.

REFERENCES

Arias, B., Catalan, R., Gasto, C., Gutierrez, B., & Fananas, L. (2005). Evidence for a combined genetic effect of the 5-HT1A receptor and serotonin transporter genes in the clinical outcome of major depressive patients treated with citalopram. *Journal of Psychopharmacology, 19*(2), 166–172.

Brüss, M., Kostanian, A., Bönisch, H., & Göthert, M. (2005). The naturally occurring Arg219Leu variant of the human 5-HT1A receptor: impairment of signal transduction. *Pharmacogenetics, 15*(4), 257–264.

Duncan, G. E., Zorn, S., & Lieberman, J. A. (1999). Mechanisms of typical and atypical antipsychotic drug action in relation to dopamine and NMDA receptor hypofunction hypotheses of schizophrenia. *Molecular Psychiatry, 4*(5), 418–428.

Glatt, C. E., Tampilic, M., Christie, C., DeYoung, J., & Freimer, N. B. (2004). Re-screening serotonin receptors for genetic variants identifies population and molecular genetic complexity. *American Journal of Medical Genetics Part B, Neuropsychiatric Genetics Genetics, 124*(1), 92–100.

Hensler, J. G. (2003). Regulation of 5-HT1A receptor function in brain following agonist or antidepressant administration. *Life Sciences, 72*(15), 1665–1682.

Invernizzi, R. W., Sacchetti, G., Parini, S., Acconcia, S., & Samanin, R. (2003). Flibanserin, a potential antidepressant drug, lowers 5-HT and raises dopamine and noradrenaline in the rat prefrontal cortex dialysate: role of 5-HT(1A) receptors. *British Journal of Pharmacology, 139*(7), 1281–1288.

Jordan, S., Koprivica, V., Chen, R., Tottori, K., Kikuchi, T., & Altar, C. A. (2002). The antipsychotic aripiprazole is a potent, partial agonist at the human 5-HT1A receptor. *European Journal of Pharmacology, 441*(3), 137–140.

Lam, S., Shen, Y., Nguyen, T., Messier, T. L., Brann, M., Comings, D., et al. (1996). A serotonin receptor gene (5HT1A) variant found in a Tourette's syndrome patient. *Biochemical & Biophysical Research Communications, 219*(3), 853–858.

Lemonde, S., Du, L., Bakish, D., Hrdina, P., & Albert, P. R. (2004). Association of the C(–1019)G 5-HT1A functional promoter polymorphism with antidepressant response. *International Journal of Neuropsychopharmacology, 7*(4), 501–506.

Lesch, K. P., & Gutknecht, L. (2004). Focus on The 5-HT1A receptor: emerging role of a gene regulatory variant in psychopathology and pharmacogenetics. *International Journal of Neuropsychopharmacology, 7*(4), 381–385.

Mrazek, D. A., O'Kane, D. J., Black, J. L., Drews, M. S., Courson, V. L., Biernacka, J. M., et al. (2008). An association of cytochrome P450 2C19 genotype and remission in patients treated with citalopram. *Biological Psychiatry, 63*(251).

Reynolds, G. P., Arranz, B., Templeman, L. A., Fertuzinhos, S., & San, L. (2006). Effect of 5-HT1A receptor gene polymorphism on negative and depressive symptom response to antipsychotic treatment of drug-naive psychotic patients. *American Journal of Psychiatry, 163*(10), 1826–1829.

Serretti, A., Artioli, P., Lorenzi, C., Pirovano, A., Tubazio, V., & Zanardi, R. (2004). The C(–1019)G polymorphism of the 5-HT1A gene promoter and antidepressant response in mood disorders: preliminary findings. *International Journal of Neuropsychopharmacology, 7*(4), 453–460.

Stark, A. D., Jordan, S., Allers, K. A., Bertekap, R. L., Chen, R., Mistry Kannan, T., et al. (2007). Interaction of the novel antipsychotic aripiprazole with

5-HT1A and 5-HT 2A receptors: functional receptor-binding and in vivo electrophysiological studies. *Psychopharmacology, 190*(3), 373–382.

Yu, Y. W., Tsai, S. J., Liou, Y. J., Hong, C. J., & Chen, T. J. (2006). Association study of two serotonin 1A receptor gene polymorphisms and fluoxetine treatment response in Chinese major depressive disorders. *European Neuropsychopharmacology, 16*(7), 498–503.

13

THE SEROTONIN 2A
RECEPTOR GENE

Variations in the serotonin 2A receptor gene (HTR2A) have been studied with the primary objective of predicting the response of patients to antidepressant medications and atypical antipsychotic medications. Although there is an extensive distribution of HTR2A receptors in the brain, concentrations of these receptors have been localized in the frontal and temporal regions.

LOCATION AND GENE VARIATION

HTR2A is located on chromosome 13. The specific location of the gene is on the long arm of chromosome 13 at 13q14-q21 (Fig. 13.1).

HTR2A consists of approximately 62,663 nucleotides or 62.7 kilobases. HTR2A contains three exons, which are composed of 3,009 nucleotides, and codes for a polypeptide composed of 471 amino acids (Chen et al., 1992) (Fig. 13.2). Interestingly, two promoters have been identified in the 5' region domain of the gene. Furthermore, a "silencer" has been identified immediately downstream from the second promoter at nucleotide location −1438 (Zhu et al., 1995). Four transcription sites have also been identified.

Table 13.1 provides a list of the most well-studied HTR2A alleles. This list includes both the ancestral and mutant alleles. Each allele is described in the following technical discussion.

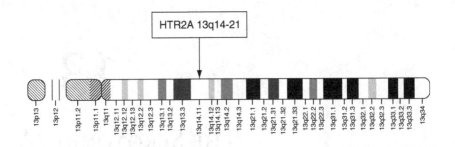

FIGURE 13.1. Chromosome 13 with arrow to designate the location of the HTR2A.

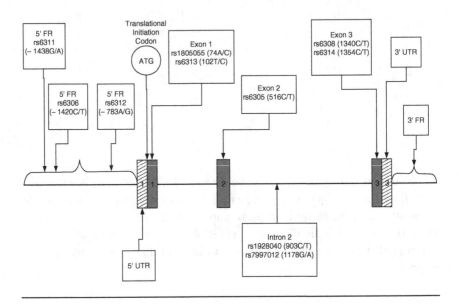

FIGURE 13.2. HTR2A structure illustrating the location of the three exons and the single nucleotide polymorphisms that define the most important HTR2A alleles.

TABLE 13.1. The locations of nucleotide changes that define the most well-studied HTR2A alleles

refSNP ID & Aliases	Nucleotide Location	Ancestral Allele	Mutant Variant
rs6311 or −1438G/A	−1438	G	A
rs6306 or −1420C/T	−1420	C	T
rs6312 or −783A/G	−783	A	G
rs1805055 or 74A/C or 5Thr/Asn	74	A	C
rs6313 or 102T/C	102	T	C
rs6305 or 516C/T	516	C	T
rs1928040 or 903C/T	903	C	T
rs7997012 or 1178G/A	1178	G	A
rs6308 or 1340C/T or 447Ala/Val	1340	C	T
rs6314 or 1354C/T or His452Tyr	1354	C	T

158

Technical Discussion of HTR2A Variations

Each of the most well-studied HTR2A alleles is described in this technical discussion.

rs6311 or –1438G/A

rs6311 is the result of an guanine to adenine change at nucleotide location –1438 in the promoter region. The adenine allele has been shown to have greater expression than the guanine allele (Parsons et al.,2004). In samples of European ancestry, there is strong to complete linkage disequilibrium between rs6311 in the promoter region and rs6313 in exon 1. The guanine allele of rs6311 is linked with the cytosine allele of rs6313. Conversely, the adenine allele of rs6311 is linked to the thymine allele of rs6313. However, in some African American samples, the linkage disequilibrium between rs6311 and rs6313 is less complete (McMahon et al., 2006).

rs6306 or –1420C/T

rs6306 is the result of a cytosine to thymine change at nucleotide location –1420 in the promoter region.

rs6312 or –783A/G

rs6312 is the result of an adenine to guanine change at nucleotide location –783 in the promoter region. An interaction between rs6312 and rs6311 has been reported. When rs6312 is the adenine allele, the activity level of the guanine allele and the adenine allele of rs6311 is similar. However, when rs6312 is the guanine allele, the expression of the adenine allele is greater than the guanine allele of rs6311 (Myers et al.,2007).

rs1805055 or 74A/C or 25Thr/Asn

rs1805055 is the result of an adenine to cytosine change at nucleotide location 74 in exon 1. This results in a change from a threonine to an asparagine at amino acid position 25 of the receptor protein (Erdman et al., 1996).

rs6313 or 102T/C

rs6313 is the result of a thymine to cytosine change at nucleotide location 102 in exon 1. In populations of European ancestry, rs6313 is in strong or complete linkage disequilibrium with rs6311. The guanine allele of rs6311 is linked with the cytosine allele of rs6313. Conversely, the adenine allele of rs6311 is linked to the thymine allele of rs6313.

rs6305 or 516C/T

rs6305 is the result of a cytosine to thymine change at nucleotide location 516 in exon 2. The thymine allele was documented to occur in less than 1% of a German sample (Erdman et al., 1996), and has been reported to be approximately 1% in other samples of European origin.

rs1928040 or 903C/T

rs1928040 is the result of a cytosine to thymine change at nucleotide location 903 in intron 2. rs1928040 is believed to be in strong linkage disequilibrium with rs6311 and rs6313 (McMahon et al., 2006).

(*Continued*)

rs7997012 or 1178G/A

rs7997012 is the result of a guanine to adenine change at nucleotide location 1178 in intron 2. rs7997012 is not in linkage disequilibrium with rs6311, rs6313, or rs1928040. Subjects who were homozygous for the adenine allele have been reported to respond more frequently to citalopram than do subjects who were homozygous for the guanine allele (McMahon et al., 2006).

rs6308 or 1340C/T or 447Ala/Val

rs6308 is the result of a cytosine to thymine change at nucleotide location 1340 in exon 3. This results in a change of an alanine to a valine at amino acid position 447. The thymine allele, which is sometimes referred to as the valine allele, occurs in about 1% of samples of European ancestry (Ozaki et al., 1996).

rs6314 or 1354C/T or His452Tyr

rs6314 is the result of a cytosine to thymine change at nucleotide location 1354 in exon 3. This results in a change of a histidine to a tyrosine at amino acid position 452. The thymine allele is far more common than the cytosine allele in most populations (Erdman et al., 1996). However, patients who are homozygous for the cytosine allele are more likely to respond to clozapine.

GENOTYPIC VARIANCE ACROSS GEOGRAPHIC ANCESTRY

In a German sample, the thymine allele of rs6313 occurred in 45% of subjects, whereas the cytosine allele occurred in 55% of the subjects (Erdman et al., 1996). However, in an Italian sample, the thymine allele was reported to occur in only about 8% (Cusin et al, 2002). In samples of European ancestry, rs6311 and rs6313 have been shown to be in strong or complete linkage disequilibrium.

In an African American sample, an association between rs6311 and a response to citalopram was demonstrated, but rs6313 did not predict a response. This association with rs6311 and citalopram response was not found in white subjects in this study (McMahon et al., 2006).

In a Korean sample of normal controls, the allele frequency of the guanine allele of rs6311 was reported to be 46%, whereas the allele frequency of the adenine allele was 54% (Choi et al., 2005). The adenine allele of rs6311 is more common in Koreans than in many samples of European ancestry.

The tyrosine variant of rs6314 (i.e., 1354C/T or His452Tyr) has been reported to have an allele frequency of about 10% in samples of European ancestry (Ozaki et al., 1996). It was not found at all in a Japanese sample (Yamanouchi et al., 2003).

ANTIDEPRESSANT MEDICATIONS

Variations in HTR2A have been associated with response to antidepressant medication, although there have been some inconsistencies in reported findings.

Citalopram

In a Korean sample, patients who were homozygous for the guanine allele of rs6311 (1438G/A) were more likely to respond to citalopram than were those patients who had an adenine allele (Choi et al., 2005). Among the subjects who were homozygous for the guanine allele, 48% fully remitted, as compared to the 30% fully remitted subjects who had one or two copies of the adenine allele. Similarly, the subjects who were homozygous for the guanine allele had 70% response rate, determined by documenting at least a 50% reduction in symptoms, compared to those with one or two copies of the adenine allele, who had a response rate of 48%.

In examining the effect of the rs7997012 (i.e., 1178G/A) adenine allele in a white sample, 80% of the subjects who were homozygous for the adenine allele were classified as responders to citalopram, compared to 64% of subjects who were homozygous for the guanine allele (McMahon et al., 2006). In this white sample, no association existed between the adenine allele of rs6311 (i.e., −1438G/A) and response to citalopram. However, there was an association between the adenine allele of rs6311 and both response to citalopram and remission of symptoms in black subjects.

Fluvoxamine and Paroxetine

Some evidence of an association between variants in HTR2A and response to fluvoxamine and paroxetine has been reported. However, these relationships are not well established. Approximately 55% of subjects who were homozygous for the cytosine allele of rs6313 (i.e., 102T/C) responded to treatment, compared to 75% of those who were homozygous for the thymine allele of rs6313. In another positive study, 65% of subjects with the cytosine allele of rs6306 (i.e., −1420C/T) responded, compared to 30% with the less common thymine allele of rs6306 (Cusin et al., 2002).

ADVERSE EFFECTS OF ANTIDEPRESSANTS

Intolerance

A study of older depressed patients reported an association between the inability to successfully continue to take paroxetine over the course of 6 weeks of treatment and having two copies of the cytosine allele of rs6313 (i.e., 102T/C). About 40% of the homozygous cytosine allele subjects discontinued paroxetine, compared to about 16% of patients with the other genotypes (Murphy et al., 2003).

Sexual Side Effects

In a sample of men and women who were taking one of a variety of selective serotonin reuptake inhibitor antidepressants, an association was reported between the guanine allele of rs6311 (i.e., −1438G/A) and sexual dysfunction. Specifically, women who were homozygous for the guanine allele of rs6311 were less likely to report having frequent sexual arousal when compared to women with other genotypes (Bishop et al., 2006).

ANTIPSYCHOTIC MEDICATIONS

Antipsychotic medications vary in their affinity to the HTR2A receptor, as illustrated in Table 13.2 (Duncan et al., 1999; Lawler et al., 1999; Stark et al., 2007).

Clozapine

In samples of European ancestry, it has been repeatedly demonstrated that the adenine allele of rs6311 (i.e., −1438G/A) and the thymine allele of rs6313 (i.e., 102T/C) are associated with a better response to clozapine than the guanine allele of rs6311 or the cytosine allele of rs6313. This finding has not been consistently demonstrated in samples of more varied ancestry. An initial report documented a response rate of 72% in patients who had one copy of the thymine allele of rs6313 that was in complete linkage disequilibrium with the adenine allele of rs6311, as compared to a response rate of 43% in patients who were homozygous for the cytosine allele of rs6313 (Arranz et al., 1995; Arranz et al., 1996; Arranz et al., 1998; Arranz et al., 2000).

TABLE 13.2. Antipsychotic drug affinity (ability to bind
to receptor) in nM

Antipsychotic Drugs	Affinity
Risperidone	High (0.29)
Ziprasidone	High (0.39)
Olanzapine	High (3.3)
Aripiprazole	High (3.4)
Clozapine	Moderate (8.9)
Haloperidol	Low (120)
Quetiapine	Low (220)

rs6314 (i.e., 1354C/T) is another variant of HTR2A that has been linked to clozapine response. rs6314 is not in strong linkage disequilibrium with either rs6311 or rs6313. Specifically, patients who had one or more copies of the very common thymine allele (i.e., histidine allele) had a response rate of 66%, whereas patients who were homozygous for the relatively rare cytosine allele (i.e., tyrosine allele) of rs6314 had a response rate of only 25% (Arranz et al., 1996).

Risperidone

A study of acutely ill Chinese patients treated with risperidone for schizophrenia reported that those who were homozygous for the cytosine allele of rs6313 (i.e., 102T/C) had more improvement in their negative symptoms than did those who carried one or more copies of the thymine allele. These patients differed from the clozapine studies in that they were more acutely ill and were of Chinese rather than European ancestry (Lane et al., 2002).

In a study of French patients, a similar association with the adenine allele of rs6311 (i.e., –1438G/A) was reported in some patients who were treated with atypical antipsychotics, including 22 subjects who received risperidone (Hamdani et al., 2005).

Olanzapine

A study of patients with schizophrenia who were primarily of European ancestry reported that those who were homozygous for the adenine allele of rs6311 (i. e. –1438G/A) experienced a 45% improvement in their negative symptoms with olanzapine, compared to a 19% improvement in negative symptoms in patients with an alternative rs6311 genotype (Ellingrod et al., 2003). A study of French patients with schizophrenia, including 51 patients who were treated with olanzapine, also reported that subjects with the adenine allele of rs6311 had more improvement in their negative symptoms (Hamdani et al., 2005).

ADVERSE EFFECTS OF ANTIPSYCHOTICS

Tardive Dyskinesia and Extrapyramidal Symptoms

Several studies have reported associations with variants of HTR2A and extrapyramidal symptoms. The cytosine allele of rs6313 (and therefore the guanine allele of rs6311) was associated with higher dyskinesia scores and more disability in a sample of Jewish ancestry with the diagnosis of chronic schizophrenia (Segman et al., 2001).

In a sample of patients with schizophrenia who were of Chinese ancestry, the cytosine allele of rs6313 was also associated with a greater likelihood of developing tardive dyskinesia (Tan et al., 2001). This same association was reported in a small sample in Estonia who were treated with the typical antipsychotic perphenazine (Gunes et al., 2007).

An Italian study also reported an association with tardive dyskinesia and the cytosine allele of rs6313 (i.e., 102T/C). In this study, 81% of patients who were homozygous for the cytosine allele of rs6313 were diagnosed with tardive dyskinesia, while 45% of patients with one or more thymine alleles of rs6313 had tardive dyskinesia (Lattuada et al., 2004).

However, in a sample of Turkish patients who were treated with antipsychotic medication, 67% of patients who were homozygous for the adenine allele of rs6311, 52% who were heterozygous for the adenine and guanine alleles of rs6311, and 38% who were homozygous for the guanine allele of rs6311 developed tardive dyskinesia (Boke et al., 2007; Lerer et al., 2005).

The analysis of a combination of data from six pharmacogenomics laboratories further supported an earlier finding that subjects with the cytosine allele of rs6313 were more likely to develop tardive dyskinesia. A haplotype composed of the cytosine allele of rs6313 and the thymine allele of rs6314 was even more predictive of tardive dyskinesia (Segman et al., 2001).

Weight Gain

Variations in both HTR2A and HTR2C (see Chapter 14) have been linked to an increased risk of weight gain when taking antipsychotic medications

(Chagnon, 2006). The adenine allele of rs6311 (i.e., −1438G/A) was associated with lower energy intake in a French population of obese patients (Aubert et al., 2000). In another study, homozygous patients with the guanine allele of rs6311 had a higher body mass index (BMI) (26.9) and a greater abdominal sagittal diameter (23.6 cm) (Rosmond et al., 2002). However, unlike variability in HTR2C, the guanine allele of rs6311 in HTR2A has not yet been shown to be predictive of weight gain secondary to treatment with antipsychotic medication.

Clinical Case 12

A 32-year-old man, whose parents were of Spanish ancestry, was diagnosed with schizophrenia. When his father developed Alzheimer disease and could no longer recognize him, the patient stopped taking his olanzapine because he felt that his recent weight gain was making it more difficult for his father to know who he was. He had been on many antipsychotic medications over the years, but he had never been treated with clozapine. His psychiatrist ordered pharmacogenomic testing (Table 13.3).

TABLE 13.3. Pharmacogenomic report of case 12

Gene	Gene Variant	Genotype	Clinical Implication
CYP2D6	N/A	*1/*2A	Extensive CYP2D6 metabolizer
CYP2C19	N/A	*1/*1	Extensive CYP2C19 metabolizer
CYP2C9	N/A	*1/*1	Extensive CYP2C9 metabolizer
CYP1A2	N/A	*1A/*1A	Extensive CYP1A2 metabolizer
COMT	rs4680	G/G	Higher Activity
SLC6A2	rs5569	G/G	Better antidepressant response
SLC6A4	Indel promoter	Long/Long	High Activity
SLC6A4	2nd intron VNTR	10-repeat/ 10-repeat	Low Activity
SLC6A4	rs25531	G/G	Low Activity
HTR2A	rs6311	A/A	Better response to clozapine
HTR2A	rs6312	G/G	Positive interaction with rs6311

His pharmacogenomic report identified several key issues that should be considered in the treatment of this relatively young patient with a well-established diagnosis of schizophrenia. The final recommendation of this report is that this patient would be a good candidate for using clozapine for multiple reasons.

The two most important genotypic findings are the genotypes for rs6311 and rs6312. This patient had a positive predictive genotype for both genes. Based on this finding alone, the patient would be predicted to have a high

(*Continued*)

likelihood of responding to clozapine (Arranz et al, 2000). However, given that the patient is also homozygous for the guanine allele of rs6312 of HTR2A, it is reasonable to conclude that he would be even more likely to respond to clozapine.

Quite independent of the HTR2A results, the patient also had a positive predictive SLC6A4 genotype. This provides further evidence that he is quite likely to have a good response. Given that he has a CYP1A2 genotype that predicts he would be an extensive metabolizer, one would be further reassured that he could tolerate clozapine at recommended doses.

KEY CLINICAL CONSIDERATIONS

- Variability in HTR2A has been associated with a differential side-effect burden to several antipsychotic medications.
- Variability in HTR2A is associated with differential response to antidepressant medications that target serotonin.
- A haplotype that includes the cytosine allele of rs6313 and the thymine allele of rs6314 is predictive of tardive dyskinesia.

REFERENCES

Arranz, M. J., Collier, D. A., Munro, J., Sham, P., Kirov, G., Sodhi, M., et al. (1996). Analysis of a structural polymorphism in the 5-HT2A receptor and clinical response to clozapine. *Neuroscience Letters, 217*(2–3), 177–178.

Arranz, M., Collier, D., Sodhi, M., Ball, D., Roberts, G., Price, J., Sham, P., & Kerwin, R. (1995). Association between clozapine response and allelic variation in 5-HT2A receptor gene. *Lancet, 346*(8970), 281–282.

Arranz, M. J., Munro, J., Birkett, J., Bolonna, A., Mancama, D. T., Sodhi, M., et al. (2000). Pharmacogenetic prediction of clozapine response. *Lancet, 355,* 1615–1616.

Arranz, M., Munro, J., Sham, P., Kirov, G., Murray, R., Collier, D., & Kerwin, R. (1998). Meta-analysis of studies on genetic variation in 5-HT2A receptors and clozapine response. *Schizophrenia Research, 32,* 93–99.

Aubert, R., Betoulle, D., Herbeth, B., Siest, G., & Fumeron, F. (2000). 5-HT2A receptor gene polymorphism is associated with food and alcohol intake in obese people. *International Journal of Obesity & Related Metabolic Disorders, 24*(7), 920–924.

Bishop, J. R., Moline, J., Ellingrod, V. L., Schultz, S. K., & Clayton, A. H. (2006). Serotonin 2A –1438 G/A and G-protein Beta3 subunit C825T polymorphisms in patients with depression and SSRI-associated sexual side-effects. *Neuropsychopharmacology, 31*(10), 2281–2288.

Boke, O., Gunes, S., Kara, N., Aker, S., Sahin, A. R., Basar, Y., & Bagci, H. (2007). Association of serotonin 2A receptor and lack of association of CYP1A2 gene polymorphism with tardive dyskinesia in a Turkish population. *DNA and cell biology, 26*(8), 527–531.

Chagnon, Y. C. (2006). Susceptibility genes for the side effect of antipsychotics on body weight and obesity. *Current Drug Targets, 7*(12), 1681–1695.

Chen, K., Yang, W., Grimsby, J., & Shih, J. C. (1992). The human 5-HT2 receptor is encoded by a multiple intron-exon gene. *Brain Research Molecular Brain Research, 14*(1–2), 20–26.

Choi, M. J., Kang, R. H., Ham, B. J., Jeong, H. Y., & Lee, M. S. (2005). Serotonin receptor 2A gene polymorphism (–1438A/G) and short-term treatment response to citalopram. *Neuropsychobiology, 52*(3), 155–162.

Cusin, C., Serretti, A., Zanardi, R., Lattuada, E., Rossini, D., Lilli, R., et al. (2002). Influence of monoamine oxidase A and serotonin receptor 2A polymorphisms in SSRI antidepressant activity. *International Journal of Neuropsychopharmacology, 5*(1), 27–35.

Duncan, G. E., Zorn, S., & Lieberman, J. A. (1999). Mechanisms of typical and atypical antipsychotic drug action in relation to dopamine and NMDA receptor hypofunction hypotheses of schizophrenia. *Molecular Psychiatry, 4*(5), 418–428.

Ellingrod, V. L., Lund, B. C., Miller, D., Fleming, F., Perry, P., Holman, T. L., & Bever-Stille, K. (2003). 5-HT2A receptor promoter polymorphism, -1438G/A and negative symptom response to olanzapine in schizophrenia. *Psychopharmacology Bulletin, 37*(2), 109–112.

Erdmann, J., Shimron-Abarbanell, D., Rietschel, M., Albus, M., Maier, W., Korner, J., et al. (1996). Systematic screening for mutations in the human serotonin-2A (5-HT2A) receptor gene: identification of two naturally occurring receptor variants and association analysis in schizophrenia. *Human Genetics, 97*(5), 614–619.

Gunes, A., Scordo, M. G., Jaanson, P., & Dahl, M. L. (2007). Serotonin and dopamine receptor gene polymorphisms and the risk of extrapyramidal side effects in perphenazine-treated schizophrenic patients. *Psychopharmacology, 190*(4), 479–484.

Hamdani, N., Bonniere, M., Ades, J., Hamon, M., Boni, C., & Gorwood, P. (2005). Negative symptoms of schizophrenia could explain discrepant data on the association between the 5-HT2A receptor gene and response to antipsychotics. *Neuroscience Letters, 377*(1), 69–74.

Lane, H. Y., Chang, Y. C., Chiu, C. C., Chen, M. L., Hsieh, M. H., & Chang, W. H. (2002). Association of risperidone treatment response with a polymorphism in the 5-HT(2A) receptor gene. *American Journal of Psychiatry, 159*(9), 1593–1595.

Lattuada, E., Cavallaro, R., Serretti, A., Lorenzi, C., & Smeraldi, E. (2004). Tardive dyskinesia and DRD2, DRD3, DRD4, 5-HT2A variants in schizophrenia: an association study with repeated assessment. *International Journal of Neuropsychopharmacology, 7*(4), 489–493.

Lawler, C. P., Prioleau, C., Lewis, M. M., Mak, C., Jiang, D., Schetz, J. A., et al. (1999). Interactions of the novel antipsychotic aripiprazole (OPC-14597) with dopamine and serotonin receptor subtypes. *Neuropsychopharmacology, 20*(6), 612–627.

Lerer, B., Segman, R. H., Tan, E. C., Basile, V. S., Cavallaro, R., Aschauer, H. N., et al. (2005). Combined analysis of 635 patients confirms an age-related association of the serotonin 2A receptor gene with tardive dyskinesia and specificity for the non-orofacial subtype. *International Journal of Neuropsychopharmacology, 8*(3), 411–425.

McMahon, F. J., Buervenich, S., Charney, D., Lipsky, R., Rush, A. J., Wilson, A. F., et al. (2006). Variation in the gene encoding the serotonin 2A receptor is associated with outcome of antidepressant treatment. *The American Journal of Human Genetics, 78*, 804–814.

Murphy, G. M., Kremer, C., Rodrigues, H. E., & Schatzberg, A. F. (2003). Pharmacogenetics of antidepressant medication intolerance. *The American Journal of Psychiatry, 160*, 1830–1835.

Myers, R. L., Airey, D. C., Manier, D. H., Shelton, R. C., & Sanders-Bush, E. (2007). Polymorphisms in the regulatory region of the human serotonin 5-HT2A receptor gene (HTR2A) influence gene expression. *Biological Psychiatry, 61*(2), 167–173.

Ozaki, N., Rosenthal, N. E., Pesonen, U., Lappalainen, J., Feldman-Naim, S., Schwartz, P. J., et al. (1996). Two naturally occurring amino acid substitutions of the 5-HT2A receptor: similar prevalence in patients with seasonal affective disorder and controls. *Biological Psychiatry, 40*(12), 1267–1272.

Parsons, M., D'Souza, U., Arranz, M., Kerwin, R., & Makoff, A. (2004). The –1438A/G Polymorphism in the 5-hydroxytryptamine type 2A receptor gene affects promoter activity. *Biological Psychiatry, 56*(6), 406–410.

Rosmond, R., Bouchard, C., & Bjorntorp, P. (2002). 5-HT2A receptor gene promoter polymorphism in relation to abdominal obesity and cortisol. *Obesity Research, 10*(7), 585–589.

Segman, R. H., Heresco-Levy, U., Finkel, B., Goltser, T., Shalem, R., Schlafman, M., et al. (2001). Association between the serotonin 2A receptor gene and tardive dyskinesia in chronic schizophrenia. *Molecular Psychiatry, 6*(2), 225–229.

Stark, A. D., Jordan, S., Allers, K. A., Bertekap, R. L., Chen, R., Mistry Kannan, T., et al. (2007). Interaction of the novel antipsychotic aripiprazole with 5-HT1A and 5-HT 2A receptors: functional receptor-binding and in vivo electrophysiological studies. *Psychopharmacology, 190*(3), 373–382.

Tan, E. C., Chong, S. A., Mahendran, R., Dong, F., & Tan, C. H. (2001). Susceptibility to neuroleptic-induced tardive dyskinesia and the T102C polymorphism in the serotonin type 2A receptor. *Biological Psychiatry, 50*(2), 144–147.

Yamanouchi, Y., Iwata, N., Suzuki, T., Kitajima, T., Ikeda, M., & Ozaki, N. (2003). Effect of DRD2, 5-HT2A, and COMT genes on antipsychotic response to risperidone. *The Pharmacogenomics Journal, 3*, 356–361.

Zhu, Q. S., Chen, K., & Shih, J. C. (1995). Characterization of the human 5-HT2A receptor gene promoter. *The Journal of Neuroscience, 15*(7), 4885–4895.

14

THE SEROTONIN 2C RECEPTOR GENE

Variations in the serotonin 2C receptor gene (HTR2C) have been associated with both response to antipsychotic medication and the occurrence of weight gain that occurs in some patients when they are treated with atypical antipsychotic medications. The distribution of HTR2C receptors in the brain includes both cortical and limbic structures.

LOCATION AND GENE VARIATION

HTR2C is located on the X chromosome. The specific location of the gene is on the long arm of the X chromosome at Xq24 (Fig. 14.1).

HTR2C consists of approximately 326,074 nucleotides or 326.1 kilobases. It contains six exons, which are composed of 4,751 nucleotides. However, HTR2C codes for a polypeptide that is composed of only 458 amino acids (Fig. 14.2).

Table 14.1 provides a list of the most well-studied HTR2C alleles and includes both the ancestral and mutant nucleotides. Each allele is described in the following technical discussion.

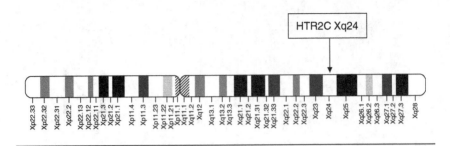

FIGURE 14.1. Chromosome X with arrow to designate the location of the HTR2C.

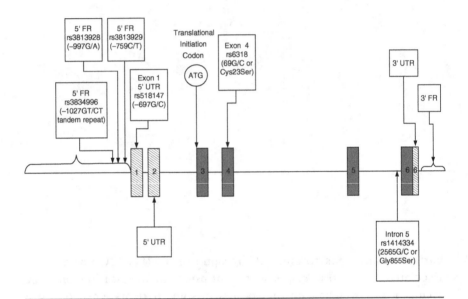

FIGURE 14.2. HTR2C structure illustrating the location of the six exons and the single nucleotide polymorphisms that define the most important HTR2C alleles.

TABLE 14.1. The locations of nucleotide changes that define the most well-studied HTR2C alleles

refSNP ID & Aliases	Nucleotide Location	Ancestral Allele	Mutant Variant
rs3834996 or −1027GT/CT tandem repeat	−1027	Short	Long
rs3813928 or −997G/A	−997	G	A
rs3813929 or −759C/T	−759	C	T
rs518147 or −697G/C	−697	G	C
rs6318 or 69G/C or Cys23Ser	69	G	C
rs1414334 or 2565G/C or Gly855Ser	2565	G[1]	C

[1]There is some controversy as to whether the G allele or the C allele is the ancestral allele.

Technical Discussion of HTR2C Variations

Each of the most well-studied HTR2C alleles is described in this technical discussion.

rs3834996 or –1027GT/CT Tandem Repeat

rs3834996 is a promoter tandem repeat polymorphism, consisting of two repeat segments. One of these is a GT-repeat segment that ranges from 12- to 18-repeats. The other is a CT-repeat segment that is either 4- or 5-repeats in length. An invariant 54 bp "spacer" exists between these two sites of variability. As a consequence of this variability, there are eight different combinations that vary in total length from 86 bp to 100 bp. Table 14.2 represents the eight possible genotypes that have been documented.

TABLE 14.2. Eight different combinations of GT- and CT-repeats make up the eight variants of rs3834996

Allele Category	Nucleotides in the GT Segment Repeat	Nucleotides in the Invariant Spacer	Nucleotides in the CT Segment Repeat	Total Number of Nucleotides that Define the Polymorphism
Short Alleles	24	54	8	86
	24	54	10	88
	28	54	8	90
	28	54	10	92
Long Alleles	32	54	8	94
	32	54	10	96
	36	54	8	98
	36	54	10	100

The 88-bp allele and the 94-bp allele are the most common alleles in patients of European ancestry. In contrast, the longest alleles (i.e., 96, 98, and 100) have a combined allelic frequency of only about 5%. For dichotomous comparisons, the four longest alleles (i.e., 94, 96, 98, and 100 alleles) are given the single classification of being the "long allele." The 88 allele is the most common allele that is classified as a "short allele" (Arranz et al., 2000). These short alleles of the variant have been described as being dominant (Deckert et al., 2000).

rs3813928 or –997G/A

rs3813928 is the result of a guanine to adenine change at nucleotide location –997 in the promoter region. rs3813928 is in relatively strong linkage disequilibrium with rs3813929 (i.e., –759C/T) (Reynolds et al., 2005a).

(*Continued*)

rs3813929 or –759C/T

rs3813929 is the result of a cytosine to thymine change at nucleotide location –759 in the promoter region. rs3813929 is in relatively strong linkage disequilibrium with rs3813928 (i.e., –997G/A) (Basile et al., 2002).

rs518147 or –697G/C

rs518147 is the result of guanine to a cytosine change at nucleotide location –697 in the promoter region. In a Chinese population, rs518147 has been reported to be in relatively strong linkage disequilibrium with rs3813929 (i.e., –759C/T) (Zhang et al., 2002).

rs6318 or 69G/C or Cys23Ser

rs6318 is the result of a guanine to cytosine change at nucleotide location 69 in exon 4. This change results in a substitution of a cysteine for a serine at amino acid position 23, which is in the extracellular N-terminal domain of the receptor (Lappalainen et al., 1995). This structural change has been associated with a change in receptor function (Sodhi et al., 1995).

rs1414334 or 2565G/C or Gly855Ser

rs1414334 is the result of a guanine to cytosine change at nucleotide location 2565 in intron 5. This change results in a glycine to serine change at amino acid position 855. Of technical interest, this change abolishes a restriction enzyme cleavage site for the restriction enzyme Hinf1. Hinf1 is an enzyme that has been derived from the *Haemophilus influenzae* bacteria. By convention, the name of the bacteria is used to create the abbreviation "Hinf1." As a consequence of the loss of the restriction enzyme cleavage site, the serine allele can be identified by using a restriction enzyme assay. This assay yields a larger 104-bp fragment if the serine allele is present or two smaller fragments of 86 bp and 18 bp if the glycine allele is present. The cytosine nucleotide must be present for the restriction enzyme to attach to the nucleotide sequence and subsequently separate the long fragment into two shorter DNA fragments (Martinez-Marignac & Bianchi, 2006; Mulder et al., 2007b).

GENOTYPIC VARIANCE ACROSS GEOGRAPHIC ANCESTRY

The most widely studied HTR2C variant is rs6318 (i.e., 69G/C or Cys23Ser). In a European sample, the ancestral cytosine allele, which codes for serine, is uniformly more common than the guanine allele, which codes for glycine. The cytosine allele frequencies ranged from 75% in a Greek sample to 91% in a Scottish sample (Lerer et al., 2001). In a separate study, the frequency of the cytosine allele was reported between 83% and 85% percent in German and Croatian populations (Stefulj et al.,

2004). In an African American sample, the cytosine allele was found to be less common than in samples of patients of European ancestry. In this sample of African ancestry, the cytosine allele frequency was about 60%, whereas in European samples the allele frequency of the cytosine allele is usually greater than 80% (Masellis et al., 1998).

A Spanish study of rs3813929 (i.e., −759C/T) reported that 67% of the women were homozygous for the cytosine allele, whereas 33% were heterozygous for the cytosine allele and the thymine allele. No women were homozygous for the rarer thymine allele. This study reported that 80% of the men carried a cytosine allele on their single X chromosome. The condition of having only one copy of a gene is described as being *hemizygous.* Consequently, 80% of the men were hemizygous for the cytosine allele, whereas 20% of the men were hemizygous for the thymine allele (Templeman et al., 2005).

ANTIDEPRESSANT MEDICATIONS

Despite HTR2C being an important serotonin receptor in the central nervous system, variance in this gene has not yet been associated with variable responses to antidepressant medications. However, antidepressants do have dramatic variation in their affinity to the HTR2C receptors. Affinity is measured by deriving a Ki value. Low Ki values reflect greater affinity. This variability in affinity has been associated with risk for weight gain (Table 14.3) (Roth & Kroeze, 2006).

TABLE 14.3. Antidepressant affinity for the HTR2C receptor

Antidepressant Drug	Affinity and Ki Value	Weight Gain Liability
Amitriptyline	High (4)	High
Mirtazapine	Moderate (8.9)	High
Fluoxetine	Low (33)	Moderate
Nefazodone	Low (72)	Low
Imipramine	Low (120)	Moderate
Duloxetine	Low (916)	Low
Citalopram	Low (300-600)	Low
Sertraline	Low (>1,000)	Low
Bupropion	Low (>10,000)	Low
Paroxetine	Low (>10,000)	Low
Venlafaxine	Low (>10,000)	Low

Ki values represent affinities either from human cloned receptors or from human brain receptors from the Ki-DB. Roth & Kroeze (2006).

ANTIPSYCHOTIC MEDICATIONS

Antipsychotic medications also have quite variable affinities to the HTR2C receptor (Table 14.4) (Duncan et al., 1999; Stark et al., 2007).

Clozapine

Clozapine is an antipsychotic medication for which variability in HTR2C has been associated with treatment response. The first evidence of an association with a better response to clozapine was reported in patients who had one or two copies of the cytosine allele (i.e., serine allele) of rs6318 (Sodhi et al., 1995). In this study, 90% of patients with the cytosine allele had a positive response to clozapine. In a subsequent report by the same research team, the combination of two variants in HTR1A and three variants of HTR2A was shown to result in a positive predictive value of 76% in a British sample (Arranz et al., 2000). A follow-up study examining the association of variability in rs6318 and response to clozapine in a heterozygous North American sample did not find a significant relationship between the cytosine allele of rs6318 and clozapine response. However, there was a positive trend for responders to have one or two copies of the cytosine allele.

Risperidone

In a Chinese sample, a study of rs3813929 (i.e., –759C/T) revealed a positive association between the cytosine allele and better response to risperidone. This positive response was entirely due to a reduction in negative symptoms (Reynolds et al., 2005b).

TABLE 14.4. Antipsychotic drug affinity to the HTR2C receptor

Antipsychotic Drugs	Affinity and Ki Value
Ziprasidone	High (0.72)
Risperidone	Moderate (10)
Olanzapine	Moderate (10)
Aripiprazole	Moderate (15)
Clozapine	Moderate (17)
Quetiapine	Low (1400)
Haloperidol	Low (4700)

Figures in parentheses represent the nM necessary to inhibit. Duncan et al. (1999); and Stark et al. (2007).

ADVERSE EFFECTS OF ANTIPSYCHOTICS

Tardive Dyskinesia

In a sample of Jewish patients, an association between the cytosine allele (i.e., serine allele) of rs6318 (i.e., 69G/C or Cys23Ser) and tardive dyskinesia has been demonstrated. However, this association was only reported in the female subjects. In this sample, 42% of the patients with tardive dyskinesia were homozygous for the guanine allele (i.e., cysteine allele) as compared to 50% of the patients who were heterozygous for the cytosine allele (i.e., serine allele) and the guanine allele (i.e., cysteine allele). Only two female patients were homozygous for the cytosine allele (i.e., serine allele), and they both developed tardive dyskinesia (Segman et al., 2000).

More recently, in a Chinese sample, the association between two promoter variants and tardive dyskinesia has been studied. The cytosine allele of rs518147 (i. e. –697G/C) was associated with increased susceptibility to dyskinesia (Zhang et al., 2002). In a small sample in Estonia who were treated with perphenazine monotherapy, the cytosine allele of rs518147 was also associated with a greater likelihood of developing tardive dyskinesia (Gunes et al., 2007).

Even more recently, in a study of an Italian sample of men with schizophrenia, the cytosine allele (i.e., serine allele) of rs6318 (i.e., 69G/C or Cys23Ser) was associated with extrapyramidal side effects. These patients were treated with classical antipsychotic medications for at least 5 years. In this study, a haplotype that included the cytosine allele was also associated with the development of extrapyramidal symptoms (Gunes et al., 2008).

Weight Gain

The cytosine allele of rs3813929 (i.e., –759C/T) has been repeatedly associated with weight gain in patients taking antipsychotic medications. In contrast, variants in the rs6318 (i.e., 69G/C or Cys23Ser) and the rs3813928 (i.e., –997G/A) have not been associated with weight gain (Chagnon, 2006).

Chinese patients who were homozygous for the cytosine allele of rs3813929 were more likely to gain weight when treated with either chlorpromazine or risperidone. In this sample, none of the patients who had at least one protective copy of the thymine allele of rs3813929 gained more than 7% of their body weight after 6 weeks of treatment. This was in contrast to 28% of the patients who did not have a protective copy of the thymine allele and who did gain more than 7% of their body weight. Later in the course of the study, after 10 weeks of treatment, 15% of the patients with one or two copies of a protective thymine allele had gained more than 7% of their body weight, while 51% of those without a copy of a protective thymine allele gained this much weight (Reynolds et al., 2002).

In a study of Spanish patients who were treated with atypical antipsychotic medications for up to 9 months, a protective effect of the thymine allele of rs3813929 was again demonstrated. This protective effect was specifically reported for those patients taking olanzapine. The thymine allele was also associated with higher levels of plasma leptin at the baseline of this study (Templeman et al., 2005). Two additional small studies of patients of European ancestry who were treated with antipsychotic medications again revealed a protective effect of the thymine allele of rs3813929 (Ellingrod et al., 2005; Miller et al., 2005).

However, in a Korean sample, the protective effect of the thymine allele of rs3813929 was not demonstrated in patients taking olanzapine (Park et al., 2008). Another study designed to replicate the protective effect of the thymine allele of rs3813929 in a sample that included patients of both European ancestry (n = 58) and African ancestry (n = 22) also did not find this association. Specifically, those patients who had a copy of the thymine allele of rs3813929 did not have less weight gain after 6 weeks of treatment with clozapine. This finding may be attributed either to the geographic ancestry of the subjects or to the choice of antipsychotic medication. Specifically, chlorpromazine or risperidone are associated with less weight gain than clozapine. An alternative explanation is that rs3813929 may be in linkage disequilibrium with another HTR2C variant and cosegregated differently in groups that vary in their geographic ancestry (Basile et al., 2002).

A meta-analysis of the association between rs3813929 variance and weight gain ultimately concluded that the thymine allele does provide some protection from weight gain. However, it is also clear that multiple factors influence weight gain and that both the ancestry of the patient and the specific antipsychotic administered must be considered (De Luca et al., 2007).

Further study of the influence of haplotypes of HTR2C on weight gain may more accurately provide estimates of risk of weight gain. One example of this strategy is a study of a haplotype that extends from nucleotide location –1027 to nucleotide location 69. A specific haplotype defined on the basis of having the long GT–repeat allele, the cytosine allele of rs3813929 (i.e., –759C/T), and the guanine allele (i.e., serine allele) of rs6318 (i.e., 69G/C or Cys23Ser), was reported to be associated with weight gain (De Luca et al., 2007) (Fig. 14.3).

Another study of HTR2C haplotypes in a European sample found an association with variants of HTR2C and weight gain and the metabolic syndrome. This study used an extended haplotype that included a fourth single nucleotide polymorphism which was rs1414334 (i.e., 2565G/C or Gly855Ser) (Mulder et al., 2007a). See Figure 14.4.

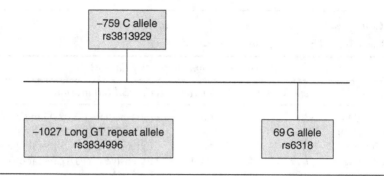

FIGURE 14.3. HTR2C haplotype associated with risk for weight gain.
De Luca et al. (2007).

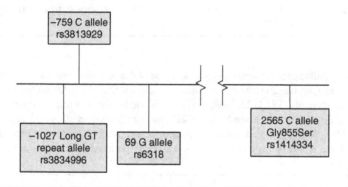

FIGURE 14.4. HTR2C haplotype associated with risk for weight gain and metabolic syndrome.
Mulder et al. (2007b).

CLINICAL IMPLICATIONS

The most compelling indication for genotyping HTR2C is to identify patients who are at increased risk for weight gain when taking atypical antipsychotic medication.

Clinical Case 13

A 54-year-old woman of Chinese ancestry had a body mass index of 31. She had a long history of chronic schizophrenia that was marked by prominent negative symptoms. She presented for psychiatric evaluation after the suicide of her daughter. At that time, her psychiatrist considered whether her treatment could be modified to increase the likelihood that she would lose weight. Pharmacogenomic testing was ordered (Table 14.5).

(*Continued*)

TABLE 14.5. Pharmacogenomic report of case 13

Gene	Gene Variant	Genotype	Clinical Implication
CYP2D6	N/A	*1/*10	Intermediate CYP2D6 metabolizer
CYP2C19	N/A	*3/*3	Poor CYP2C19 metabolizer
CYP2C9	N/A	*1/*1	Extensive CYP2C9 metabolizer
CYP1A2	N/A	*1A/*1F	Extensive CYP1A2 metabolizer
COMT	rs4680	A/A	Lower Activity
SLC6A2	rs5569	G/G	Better antidepressant response
SLC6A4	rs4495541	Short/Short	Lower Activity
HTR1A	rs6295	C/C	Better response to clozapine
HTR2A	rs6311	A/A	Better response to clozapine
HTR2C	rs6318	C/C	Better response to clozapine
HTR2C	rs3813929	T/T	Less weight gain risk

A key finding in the pharmacogenomic report of this patient is that she is at lower risk for weight gain using clozapine or risperidone, given that she is homozygous for the thymine allele of rs3813929. However, risperidone would be a more difficult drug to manage for this patient, given her poor 2D6 metabolizer status. Although clozapine is more likely to be effective because the patient is homozygous for the cytosine allele of rs6318, the risk of agranulocytosis must also be considered in deciding on the use of clozapine.

KEY CLINICAL CONSIDERATION

- The cytosine allele of rs3813929 (i.e., −759C/T) has consistently been associated with an increased risk for weight gain. Particular caution should be exercised in prescribing atypical antipsychotic medications that have been demonstrated to stimulate weight gain in patients who do not have a copy of the protective thymine allele.

REFERENCES

Arranz, M. J., Munro, J., Birkett, J., Bolonna, A., Mancama, D. T., Sodhi, M., et al. (2000). Pharmacogenetic prediction of clozapine response. *Lancet, 355*, 1615–1616.

Basile, V. S., Masellis, M., De Luca, V., Meltzer, H. Y., & Kennedy, J. L. (2002). −759C/T genetic variation of 5HT(2C) receptor and clozapine-induced weight gain. *Lancet, 360*(9347), 1790–1791.

Chagnon, Y. C. (2006). Susceptibility genes for the side effect of antipsychotics on body weight and obesity. *Current Drug Targets, 7*(12), 1681–1695.

De Luca, V., Muller, D. J., Hwang, R., Lieberman, J. A., Volavka, J., Meltzer, H. Y., & Kennedy, J. L. (2007). HTR2C haplotypes and antipsychotics-induced weight gain: X-linked multimarker analysis. *Human Psychopharmacology, 22*(7), 463–467.

Deckert, J., Meyer, J., Catalano, M., Bosi, M., Sand, P., DiBella, D., et al. (2000). Novel 5'-regulatory region polymorphisms of the 5-HT2C receptor gene: association study with panic disorder. *The International Journal of Neuropsychopharmacology: Official Scientific Journal of the Collegium Internationale Neuropsychopharmacologicum (CINP), 3*(4), 321–325.

Duncan, G. E., Zorn, S., & Lieberman, J. A. (1999). Mechanisms of typical and atypical antipsychotic drug action in relation to dopamine and NMDA receptor hypofunction hypotheses of schizophrenia. *Molecular Psychiatry, 4*(5), 418–428.

Ellingrod, V. L., Perry, P. J., Ringold, J. C., Lund, B. C., Bever-Stille, K., Fleming, F., et al. (2005). Weight gain associated with the –759C/T polymorphism of the 5HT2C receptor and olanzapine. *American Journal of Medical Genetics Part B, Neuropsychiatric Genetics: The Official Publication of the International Society of Psychiatric Genetics, 134*(1), 76–78.

Gunes, A., Dahl, M. L., Spina, E., & Scordo, M. G. (2008). Further evidence for the association between 5-HT2C receptor gene polymorphisms and extrapyramidal side effects in male schizophrenic patients. *European Journal of Clinical Pharmacology, 64*(5), 477–482.

Gunes, A., Scordo, M. G., Jaanson, P., & Dahl, M. L. (2007). Serotonin and dopamine receptor gene polymorphisms and the risk of extrapyramidal side effects in perphenazine-treated schizophrenic patients. *Psychopharmacology, 190*(4), 479–484.

Lappalainen, J., Zhang, L., Dean, M., Oz, M., Ozaki, N., Yu, D., et al. (1995). Identification, expression, and pharmacology of a Cys23-Ser23 substitution in the human 5-HT2C receptor gene (HTR2C). *Genomics, 27*(2), 274–279.

Lerer, B., Macciardi, F., Segman, R. H., Adolfsson, R., Blackwood, D., Blairy, S., et al. (2001). Variability of 5-HT2C receptor cys23ser polymorphism among European populations and vulnerability to affective disorder. *Molecular Psychiatry, 6*(5), 579–585.

Martinez-Marignac, V. L., & Bianchi, N. O. (2006). Prevalence of dopamine and 5HT2C receptor polymorphisms in Amerindians and in an urban population from Argentina. *American Journal of Human Biology, 18*(6), 822–828.

Masellis, M., Basile, V., Meltzer, H. Y., Lieberman, J. A., Sevy, S., Macciardi, F. M., et al. (1998). Serotonin subtype 2 receptor genes and clinical response to clozapine in schizophrenia patients. *Neuropsychopharmacology, 19*(2), 123–132.

Miller, D. D., Ellingrod, V. L., Holman, T. L., Buckley, P. F., & Arndt, S. (2005). Clozapine-induced weight gain associated with the 5HT2C receptor –759C/T polymorphism. *American Journal of Medical Genetics Part B, Neuropsychiatric Genetics, 133*(1), 97–100.

Mulder, H., Franke, B., van der-Beek van der, A. A., Arends, J., Wilmink, F. W., Egberts, A. C., & Scheffer, H. (2007a). The association between HTR2C polymorphisms and obesity in psychiatric patients using antipsychotics: a cross-sectional study. *Pharmacogenomics Journal, 7*(5), 318–324.

Mulder, H., Franke, B., van der-Beek van der, A. A., Arends, J., Wilmink, F. W., Scheffer, H., & Egberts, A. C. (2007b). The association between HTR2C gene polymorphisms and the metabolic syndrome in patients with schizophrenia. *Journal of Clinical Psychopharmacology, 27*(4), 338–343.

Park, Y. M., Cho, J. H., Kang, S. G., Choi, J. E., Lee, S. H., Kim, L., & Lee, H. J. (2008). Lack of association between the –759C/T polymorphism of the 5-HT2C receptor gene and olanzapine-induced weight gain among Korean schizophrenic patients. *Journal of Clinical Pharmacy & Therapeutics, 33*(1), 55–60.

Reynolds, G. P., Templeman, L. A., & Zhang, Z. J. (2005a). The role of 5-HT2C receptor polymorphisms in the pharmacogenetics of antipsychotic drug treatment. *Progress in Neuro-Psychopharmacology & Biological Psychiatry, 29*(6), 1021–1028.

Reynolds, G. P., Yao, Z., Zhang, X., Sun, J., & Zhang, Z. (2005b). Pharmacogenetics of treatment in first-episode schizophrenia: D3 and 5-HT2C receptor polymorphisms separately associate with positive and negative symptom response. *European Neuropsychopharmacology, 15*(2), 143–151.

Reynolds, G. P., Zhang, Z. J., & Zhang, X. B. (2002). Association of antipsychotic drug-induced weight gain with a 5-HT2C receptor gene polymorphism. *Lancet, 359*(9323), 2086–2087.

Roth, B. L., & Kroeze, W. K. (2006). Screening the receptorome yields validated molecular targets for drug discovery. *Current Pharmaceutical Design, 12*(14), 1785–1795.

Segman, R. H., Heresco-Levy, U., Finkel, B., Inbar, R., Neeman, T., Schlafman, M., et al. (2000). Association between the serotonin 2C receptor gene and tardive dyskinesia in chronic schizophrenia: additive contribution of 5-HT2Cser and DRD3gly alleles to susceptibility. *Psychopharmacology, 152*(4), 408–413.

Sodhi, M. S., Arranz, M. J., Curtis, D., Ball, D. M., Sham, P., Roberts, G. W., et al. (1995). Association between clozapine response and allelic variation in the 5-HT2C receptor gene. *Neuroreport, 7*(1), 169–172.

Stark, A. D., Jordan, S., Allers, K. A., Bertekap, R. L., Chen, R., Mistry Kannan, T., et al. (2007). Interaction of the novel antipsychotic aripiprazole with 5-HT1A and 5-HT 2A receptors: functional receptor-binding and in vivo electrophysiological studies. *Psychopharmacology, 190*(3), 373–382.

Stefulj, J., Buttner, A., Kubat, M., Zill, P., Balija, M., Eisenmenger, W., et al. (2004). 5HT-2C receptor polymorphism in suicide victims. Association studies in German and Slavic populations. *European Archives of Psychiatry & Clinical Neuroscience, 254*(4), 224–227.

Templeman, L. A., Reynolds, G. P., Arranz, B., & San, L. (2005). Polymorphisms of the 5-HT2C receptor and leptin genes are associated with antipsychotic drug-induced weight gain in Caucasian subjects with a first-episode psychosis. *Pharmacogenetics & Genomics, 15*(4), 195–200.

Zhang, Z. J., Zhang, X. B., Sha, W. W., Zhang, X. B., & Reynolds, G. P. (2002). Association of a polymorphism in the promoter region of the serotonin 5-HT2C receptor gene with tardive dyskinesia in patients with schizophrenia. *Molecular Psychiatry, 7*(7), 670–671.

VI

THE DOPAMINE RECEPTOR GENES

15

THE DOPAMINE D2 RECEPTOR GENE

The dopamine receptor 2 gene (DRD2) has eight variants that are associated with predicting either the therapeutic response to antipsychotic medications or the side-effect liability associated with these medications. Dopamine 2 (D2) receptors are primarily located in the substantia nigra and the ventral tegmental area, although they are also located in the caudate, putamen, nucleus accumbens, and the olfactory tubercle (Mengod et al., 1992). Despite extensive research, widespread utilization of clinical genotyping of the DRD2 gene has not yet been generally implemented.

LOCATION AND GENE VARIATION

DRD2 is located on chromosome 11. The specific location of the gene is on the long arm of chromosome 11 at 11q23 (Fig. 15.1).

DRD2 consists of approximately 65,565 nucleotides or 65.6 kilobases. It contains eight exons, composed of 2,579 nucleotides. However, there is some uncertainty about the consistency of some of these coding regions. DRD2 codes for a polypeptide that is composed of 443 amino acids (Fig. 15.2) that can be organized to form two molecularly distinct proteins. The short form is designated as D2S and the long form is referred to as D2L (Picetti et al., 1997). D2L contains 29 more amino acids than D2S. The location of these additional amino acids is in the third intracellular loop of the polypeptide (Usiello et al., 2000).

Table 15.1 provides a list of the most well-studied DRD2 alleles and includes both the ancestral and mutant nucleotides. Each allele is described in the following technical discussion.

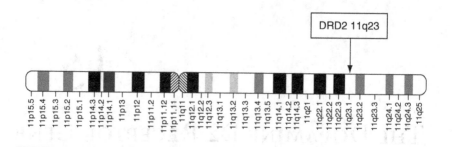

FIGURE 15.1. Chromosome 11 with arrow to designate the location of the DRD2.

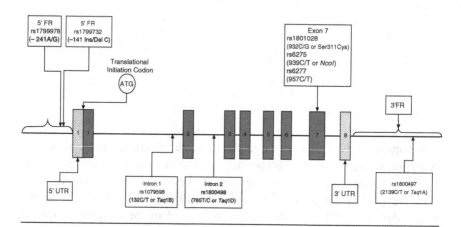

FIGURE 15.2. DRD2 structure illustrating the location of the eight exons and the single nucleotide polymorphisms that define the most important DRD2 alleles.

TABLE 15.1. The locations of nucleotide changes that define the most well-studied DRD2 alleles

refSNP ID & Aliases	Nucleotide Location	Ancestral Allele	Mutant Variant
rs1799978 or -241A/G	−241	A	G
rs1799732 or -141 Ins/Del C	−141	C	Deletion of C
rs1079598 or 132C/T or Taq1B	132	C	T
rs1800498 or 765T/C or Taq1D	765	T	C
rs1801028 or 932C/G or Ser311Cys	932	C	G
rs6275 or 939C/T or NcoI	939	C	T
rs6277 or 957C/T	957	C	T
rs1800497 or 2139C/T or Taq1A[1]	2139	C	T

[1] rs1800497 has been recently demonstrated to also be located in an overlapping gene, ankyrin repeat and kinase domain containing 1 (ANKKI)

Technical Discussion of DRD2 Variations

Each of the most well-studied DRD2 alleles is described in this technical discussion.

rs1799978 or –241A/G

rs1799978 is the result of an adenine to guanine change at nucleotide location –241 in the promoter region.

rs1799732 or –141 Ins/Del C

rs1799732 is the result of a deletion of a cytosine at nucleotide location –141 in the promoter region.

rs1079598 or 132C/T or *Taq*1B

rs1079598 is the result of a cytosine to thymine change at nucleotide location 132 in intron 1. rs1079598 was initially described as *Taq*1B, as it was originally identified using the *Taq*1 restriction fragment enzyme. The two alleles were originally referred to as the B1 allele and the B2 allele. The B1 allele refers to the cytosine allele and the B2 allele refers to the thymine allele (Hwang et al., 2005).

rs1800498 or 765T/C or *Taq*1D

rs1800498 is the result of a thymine to cytosine change at nucleotide location 765 in intron 2. rs1800498 was initially described as *Taq*1D, as it was originally identified using the *Taq*1 restriction fragment enzyme.

rs1801028 or 932C/G or Ser311Cys

rs1801028 is the result of a cytosine to guanine change at nucleotide location 932 in exon 7. This change results in an amino acid change from a serine to a cysteine at amino acid position 311, which lies in the middle portion of the third intracellular loop of the short form of DRD2 (Lane et al., 2004).

rs6275 or 939C/T or *Nco*I

rs6275 is the result of a cytosine to thymine change at nucleotide location 939 in exon 7. rs6275 was initially described as *Nco*I, as it was originally identified using the *Nco*I restriction fragment enzyme.

rs6277 or 957C/T

rs6277 is the result of a cytosine to thymine change at nucleotide location 957 in exon 7. rs6277 is in moderate linkage disequilibrium with rs1799732 (i.e., –141 indel C) and rs1800497 (i.e., *Taq*1A) (Duan et al., 2003).

rs1800497 or 2139C/T or *Taq*1A

rs1800497 is the result of a cytosine to thymine change at nucleotide location 2139 in intron 8. rs1800497 was initially described as *Taq*1A, as it was originally identified using the *Taq* restriction fragment enzyme. Originally, the two alleles were referred to as the A1 allele and the A2 allele. The A1 allele of rs1800497 (i.e., *Taq*1A) is the thymine allele and is quite rare in some populations (Makoff et al., 2000). The A2 allele of rs1800497 is the cytosine allele. rs1800497 has been recently demonstrated to also be located in an overlapping gene, ankyrin repeat and kinase domain containing 1 (ANKKI).

GENOTYPIC VARIANCE IN POPULATIONS OF DIFFERENT GEOGRAPHIC ANCESTRY

Little systematic genotypic variance has been described across groups of different geographic ancestry. However, different allelic frequencies for rs1800497 (i.e., *Taq*1A) and rs1079598 (i.e., *Taq*1B) in European versus African American samples have been reported (Hwang et al., 2005). The thymine allele (i.e., A1) of rs1800497 (i.e., *Taq*1A) has been reported to occur in 9% of some African American samples (Duan et al., 2003) and in 19% in a sample of patients of European ancestry (Hwang et al., 2005). In contrast, the thymine allele of rs1800497 has been reported to be more common in South American samples, where it occurs in 42% of Amerindians (Martinez-Marignac, et al., 2006).

ANTIDEPRESSANT MEDICATIONS

Bupropion

Variants of DRD2 have not been clearly associated with either response to antidepressant medications or adverse effects to most antidepressants. However, positive bupropion response, when used for the treatment of nicotine addiction, has been demonstrated in patients who are homozygous for the allele of rs1799732 (i.e., –141 Ins/Del C), which does not have a deleted cytosine (Lerman et al., 2006). A positive response was also noted in patients who are homozygous for the cytosine allele (i.e., the A2 allele) of rs1800497 (i.e., *Taq*1A) when compared to other rs1800497 genotypes (David et al., 2003).

ANTIPSYCHOTIC MEDICATIONS

Wide variability in the affinity of antipsychotic medications to the D2 receptor has been reported as illustrated in Table 15.2. Affinity refers to the ability of a drug to bind to a receptor. The affinity of clozapine and quetiapine to the D2 receptor is relatively low, whereas the affinity of risperidone, aripiprazole, and haloperidol to the D2 receptor is rather high.

Risperidone and Chlorpromazine

Three independent associations have been reported between DRD2 variants and antipsychotic response. The adenine allele of rs1799978 (i.e., –241A/G)

TABLE 15.2. Antipsychotic drug affinity for DRD2 receptors in nM

Antipsychotic Drugs	D2 Receptor Affinity (nM)
Risperidone	High (2.2)
Aripiprazole	High (2.4)
Haloperidol	High (2.5)
Ziprasidone	Moderate (7.2)
Olanzapine	Low (20)
Clozapine	Low (130)
Quetiapine	Low (940)

Duncan et al. (1999); and Lawler et al. (1999).

has been reported to be associated with a more rapid response to risperidone when compared to the guanine allele (Xing et al., 2007). Similarly, patients with a copy of the guanine allele of rs1801028 (i.e., 932C/G or Ser311Cys) have been reported to respond more rapidly to risperidone when compared to patients who were homozygous for the more common cytosine allele (Lane et al., 2004). Finally, patients without the cytosine allele of rs1799732 (i.e., −141 Ins/Del C) had a more rapid response to chlorpromazine than did patients who carried an allele with a deleted cytosine (Wu et al., 2005).

ADVERSE EFFECTS OF ANTIPSYCHOTICS

Tardive Dyskinesia and Extrapyramidal Side Effects

In a small study of European patients, an association has been reported between homozygosity of the cytosine allele (i.e., A2) of rs1800497 (i.e., Taq1A) and the development of dyskinesia. Four of 11 patients (36%) with two copies of the cytosine allele developed symptoms of movement disorder (Dahmen et al., 2001). This finding was replicated and extended by demonstrating that the combination of homozygosity of the cytosine allele (i.e., A2/A2) of rs1800497 (i.e., Taq 1A) and homozygosity of the thymine allele (i.e., B2/B2) of rs1079598 (i.e., Taq1B) was associated with increased risk of tardive dyskinesia. A haplotype composed of the cytosine allele (i.e., A2) of rs1800497 (i.e., Taq 1A) and the thymine allele (i.e., B2) of rs1079598 (i.e., Taq 1B) was associated with lower risk of tardive dyskinesia (Liou et al., 2006). In a third independent study of European patients, the cytosine allele (i.e., A2) of rs1800497 (i.e., Taq1A) was associated with higher risk for the development of tardive dyskinesia (Zai et al., 2007).

Neuroleptic Malignant Syndrome

Patients with schizophrenia who have a genotype that includes the deleted cytosine allele of rs1799732 (i.e., –141 Ins/Del C) have been reported to be at greater risk for neuroleptic malignant syndrome (Kishida et al., 2004; Mihara et al., 2003).

Weight Gain

Obesity has been shown to occur more frequently in patients who are homozygous for the thymine allele (i.e., A1 allele) of rs1800497 (i.e., *Taq*1A) when compared to individuals who have one or two copies of the cytosine allele (Stice et al., 2008). The thymine allele is proposed to be associated with decreased function of the D2 receptor in the striatum, and this may lead patients to continue to eat in an attempt to compensate for a decreased perception of pleasure or satiety.

CLINICAL IMPLICATIONS

Although clinical genotyping of the DRD2 gene has not been extensively implemented, the potential clearly exists for the identification of variants that place patients at increased risk for side effects when taking antipsychotic medications. Clinical Case 14 illustrates this potential clinical application.

Clinical Case 14

A 23-year-old woman had achieved considerable recognition as a talented actress when she unexpectedly experienced an acute psychotic break after having taken a large dose of LSD while traveling to London for a weekend opening of a new play at the National Theatre. Her maternal uncle had been diagnosed with bipolar disorder, and her paternal grandmother had been institutionalized in a state psychiatric hospital with a poorly understood psychotic condition characterized by paranoid delusions. Her psychiatrist felt it was clinically indicated that she receive an antipsychotic medication, but the patient was terrified of gaining weight. Pharmacogenomic testing was ordered (Table 15.3.).

The patient's pharmacogenomic report indicated that her homozygous cytosine allele (i.e., A2) of rs1800497 (i.e., Taq1A) for DRD2 and her homozygous thymine allele of rs3813929 (i.e., –759C/T) for HTR2C were both associated with a decreased risk for weight gain when treated with atypical antipsychotic medication. Given the patient's concern about gaining weight, her psychiatrist suggested that she take aripiprazole. He also felt confident that she could tolerate a standard dose of this medication, given that she was an

TABLE 15.3. Pharmacogenomic report of case 14

Pharmacogenomic Report of Case 14			
Gene	Gene Variant	Genotype	Clinical Implication
CYP2D6	N/A	*1/*2A	Extensive CYP2D6 metabolizer
CYP2C19	N/A	*1/*1	Extensive CYP2C19 metabolizer
CYP2C9	N/A	*3/*3	Poor CYP2C9 metabolizer
CYP1A2	N/A	*1F/*1F	Extensive CYP1A2 metabolizer
COMT	rs4680	G/G	Higher Activity
SLC6A4	Indel promoter	Short/Short	Lower Activity
HTR2A	rs6311	A/A	Better antipsychotic response
HTR2C	rs3813929	T/T	Less risk of weight gain
DRD2	rs1800497	C/C	Less risk of weight gain

extensive CYP2D6 metabolizer. The patient was reassured by her pharmacogenomic genotyping results, as they provided her some evidence-based support that she would have a higher probability of being able to control her weight while receiving effective treatment.

KEY CLINICAL CONSIDERATIONS

- The guanine allele of rs1801028 (i.e., 932C/G or Ser311Cys) may be associated with a better response to antipsychotic medication.
- The cytosine allele of rs1800497 (i.e., Taq1A) may be associated with decreased risk of weight gain in patients treated with antipsychotic medication.
- Schizophrenic patients who have the deleted allele of rs1799732 (i.e., −141 Ins/Del C) may be at greater risk for the neuroleptic malignant syndrome.

REFERENCES

Dahmen, N., Muller, M. J., Germeyer, S., Rujescu, D., Anghelescu, I., Hiemke, C., & Wetzel, H. (2001). Genetic polymorphisms of the dopamine D_2 and D_3 receptor and neuroleptic drug effects in schizophrenic patients. *Schizophrenia Research, 49*(1–2), 223–225.

David, S. P., Niaura, R., Papandonatos, G. D., Shadel, W. G., Burkholder, G. J., Britt, D. M., et al. (2003). Does the DRD2-Taq1 A polymorphism influence treatment response to bupropion hydrochloride for reduction of the nicotine withdrawal syndrome? *Nicotine & Tobacco Research, 5*(6), 935–942.

Duan, J., Wainwright, M. S., Comeron, J. M., Saitou, N., Sanders, A. R., Gelernter, J., & Gejman, P. V. (2003). Synonymous mutations in the human dopamine receptor D_2 (DRD2) affect mRNA stability and synthesis of the receptor. *Human Molecular Genetics, 12*(3), 205–216.

Duncan, G. E., Zorn, S., & Lieberman, J. A. (1999). Mechanisms of typical and atypical antipsychotic drug action in relation to dopamine and NMDA receptor hypofunction hypotheses of schizophrenia. *Molecular Psychiatry, 4*(5), 418–428.

Hwang, R., Shinkai, T., De Luca, V., Muller, D. J., Ni, X., Macciardi, F., et al. (2005). Association study of 12 polymorphisms spanning the dopamine D(2) receptor gene and clozapine treatment response in two treatment refractory/intolerant populations. *Psychopharmacology, 181*(1), 179–187.

Kishida, I., Kawanishi, C., Furuno, T., Kato, D., Ishigami, T., & Kosaka, K. (2004). Association in Japanese patients between neuroleptic malignant syndrome and functional polymorphisms of the dopamine D(2) receptor gene. *Molecular Psychiatry, 9*(3), 293–298.

Lane, H. Y., Lee, C. C., Chang, Y. C., Lu, C. T., Huang, C. H., & Chang, W. H. (2004). Effects of dopamine D_2 receptor Ser311Cys polymorphism and clinical factors on risperidone efficacy for positive and negative symptoms and social function. *International Journal of Neuropsychopharmacology, 7*(4), 461–470.

Lawler, C. P., Prioleau, C., Lewis, M. M., Mak, C., Jiang, D., Schetz, J. A., et al. (1999). Interactions of the novel antipsychotic aripiprazole (OPC-14597) with dopamine and serotonin receptor subtypes. *Neuropsychopharmacology, 20*(6), 612–627.

Lerman, C., Jepson, C., Wileyto, E. P., Epstein, L. H., Rukstalis, M., Patterson, F., et al. (2006). Role of functional genetic variation in the dopamine D_2 receptor (DRD2) in response to bupropion and nicotine replacement therapy for tobacco dependence: results of two randomized clinical trials. *Neuropsychopharmacology, 31*(1), 231–242.

Liou, Y. J., Lai, I. C., Liao, D. L., Chen, J. Y., Lin, C. C., Lin, C. Y., et al. (2006). The human dopamine receptor D_2 (DRD2) gene is associated with tardive dyskinesia in patients with schizophrenia. *Schizophrenia Research, 86*(1–3), 323–325.

Makoff, A., Graham, J., Arranz, M., Forsyth, J., Li, T., Aitchison, K., Shaikh, S., & Grunewald, R. (2000). Association study of dopamine receptor gene polymorphisms with drug-induced hallucinations in patients with idiopathic Parkinson's disease. *Pharmacogenetics, 10*, 43–48.

Martinez-Marignac, V. L., & Bianchi, N. O. (2006). Prevalence of dopamine and 5HT2C receptor polymorphisms in Amerindians and in an urban population from Argentina. *American Journal of Human Biology, 18*(6), 822–828.

Mengod, G., Villaro, M. T., Landwehrmeyer, G. B., Martinez-Mir, M. I., Niznik, H. B., Sunahara, R. K., et al. (1992). Visualization of dopamine D1, D_2 and D_3 receptor mRNAs in human and rat brain. *Neurochemistry International, 20 Suppl*, 33S–43S.

Mihara, K., Kondo, T., Suzuki, A., Yasui-Furukori, N., Ono, S., Sano, A., et al. (2003). Relationship between functional dopamine D_2 and D_3 receptors gene polymorphisms and neuroleptic malignant syndrome. *American Journal of Medical Genetics Part B, Neuropsychiatric Genetics: The Official Publication of the International Society of Psychiatric Genetics, 117B*(1), 57–60.

Picetti, R., Saiardi, A., Abdel Samad, T., Bozzi, Y., Baik, J. H., & Borrelli, E. (1997). Dopamine D$_2$ receptors in signal transduction and behavior. *Critical Reviews in Neurobiology 11*(2–3), 121–142.

Stice, E., Spoor, S., Bohon, C., & Small, D. M. (2008). Relation between obesity and blunted striatal response to food is moderated by TaqIA A1 allele. *Science, 322*(5900), 449–452.

Usiello, A., Baik, J. H., Rouge-Pont, F., Picetti, R., Dierich, A., LeMeur, M., et al. (2000). Distinct functions of the two isoforms of dopamine D$_2$ receptors. *Nature, 408*(6809), 199–203.

Wu, S., Xing, Q., Gao, R., Li, X., Gu, N., Feng, G., & He, L. (2005). Response to chlorpromazine treatment may be associated with polymorphisms of the DRD2 gene in Chinese schizophrenic patients. *Neuroscience Letters, 376*(1), 1–4.

Xing, Q., Qian, X., Li, H., Wong, S., Wu, S., Feng, G., et al. (2007). The relationship between the therapeutic response to risperidone and the dopamine D$_2$ receptor polymorphism in Chinese schizophrenia patients. *International Journal of Neuropsychopharmacology, 10*(5), 631–637.

Zai, C. C., De Luca, V., Hwang, R. W., Voineskos, A., Muller, D. J., Remington, G., & Kennedy, J. L. (2007). Meta-analysis of two dopamine D$_2$ receptor gene polymorphisms with tardive dyskinesia in schizophrenia patients. *Molecular Psychiatry, 12*(9), 794–795.

16

THE DOPAMINE D3 RECEPTOR GENE

The dopamine D3 receptor gene (DRD3) codes for the dopamine D3 receptor, which is pharmacologically similar to the dopamine D2 receptor. However, DRD3 is primarily expressed in the limbic region of the striatum (Joyce, 2001). Most of the pharmacogenomics research involving the DRD3 gene has examined how variations in structure have influenced therapeutic response to antipsychotic medications, as well as the adverse effects of these medications.

LOCATION AND GENE VARIATION

DRD3 is located on chromosome 3. The specific location of the gene is on the long arm of chromosome 3 at 3q13.3 (Fig. 16.1).

DRD3 consists of approximately 50,343 nucleotides or 50.3 kilobases. It contains eight exons, which are composed of 1,541 nucleotides. DRD3 codes for a polypeptide that is composed of 367 amino acids (Fig. 16.2).

Table 16.1 provides a list of the most important DRD3 alleles and includes both the ancestral and mutant nucleotides. Each allele is described in the following technical discussion.

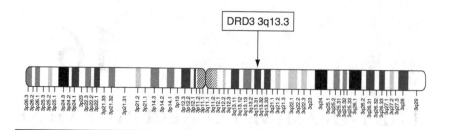

FIGURE 16.1. Chromosome 3 with arrow to designate the location of the DRD3.

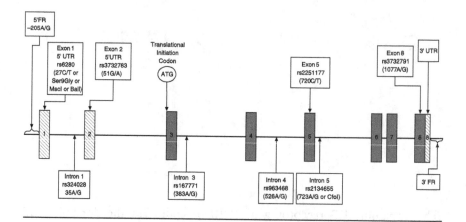

FIGURE 16.2. DRD3 structure illustrating the location of the eight exons and the single nucleotide polymorphisms that define the most important DRD3 alleles.

TABLE 16.1. The locations of nucleotide changes that define the most well-studied DRD3 alleles

refSNP ID & Aliases	Nucleotide Location	Ancestral Allele	Mutant Variant
rs (number unknown) or -205A/G	−205	A	G
rs6280 or 27C/T or Ser9Gly or MscI or BalI	27	C	T
rs324028 or 35A/G	35	A	G
rs3732783 or 51G/A	51	G	A
rs167771 or 383A/G	383	A	G
rs963468 or 526A/G	526	A	G
rs2251177 or 720C/T	720	C	T
rs2134655 or 723A/G	723	A	G
rs3732791 or 1077A/G	1077	A	G

Technical Discussion of DRD3 Variations

Each of the most well-studied DRD3 alleles is described in this technical discussion.

rs (Number Unknown) or –205A/G

–205A/G is the result of an adenine to guanine change at nucleotide location –205 in the promoter region.

rs6280 or 27C/T or Ser9Gly or MscI or BalI

rs6280 is the result of a cytosine to thymine change at nucleotide location 27 in exon 1. This change results in an amino acid change from a serine to a glycine in the N-terminal part of the receptor at amino acid position 9.

rs324028 or 35A/G

rs324028 is the result of an adenine to guanine change at nucleotide location 35 in intron 1.

rs3732783 or 51G/A

rs3732783 is the result of a guanine to adenine change at nucleotide location 51 exon 2.

rs167771 or 383A/G

rs167771 is the result of an adenine to guanine change at nucleotide location 383 in intron 3.

rs963468 or 526A/G

rs963468 is the result of an adenine to guanine change at nucleotide location 526 in intron 4.

rs2251177 or 720C/T

rs2251177 is the result of a cytosine to thymine change at nucleotide location 720 in exon 5.

rs2134655 or 723A/G

rs2134655 is the result of an adenine to guanine change at nucleotide location 723 in intron 5. rs2134655 is in considerable, but not complete, linkage disequilibrium with rs6280. This SNP also alters a CfoI restriction enzyme site (Adams et al., 2008).

rs3732791 or 1077A/G

rs3732791 is the result of an adenine to guanine change at nucleotide location 1077 in exon 8.

GENOTYPIC VARIANCE ACROSS GEOGRAPHIC ANCESTRY

Variation in geographic ancestry of rs6280 (i.e., Ser9Gly) has been the most widely studied DRD3 polymorphism. In most samples, the cytosine allele (i.e., serine allele) is the most frequent (Ma et al., 2008). The cytosine allele of rs6280 was reported to be as high as 76% in a Japanese sample and 75% in an Italian sample. The lowest reported allele frequency of the cytosine allele of rs6280 has been 52%, which was found in both a Portuguese sample and an Indian sample.

A study of Chinese patients with schizophrenia reported that the allele frequency of the cytosine allele (i.e., serine allele) of rs6280 was 68% (Xuan et al., 2008). This study also reported that the allele frequency of the adenine allele of rs324028 was 69% and that the allele frequency of the guanine allele of rs2134655 was 76%.

A study of South American populations reported the widest variability in allele frequencies. The allele frequency of the cytosine allele (i.e., serine allele) of rs6280 (i.e., Ser9Gly) was reported to be 83% in a Pehuenches population. In contrast, in a Mataco-Mataguayos population, the allele frequency of the cytosine allele of rs6280 was reported to be 38% (Martinez-Marignac & Bianchi, 2006).

ANTIDEPRESSANT MEDICATIONS

No consistent associations between genetic variability in DRD3 and anti-depressant response or adverse effects have been established.

ANTIPSYCHOTIC MEDICATIONS

A number of studies have examined variation in rs6280 (i.e., Ser9Gly) and response to antipsychotic medication. The cytosine allele (i.e., serine allele) has been associated with a more positive response to typical antipsychotic medication (Scharfetter, 2004), whereas the thymine allele (i.e., glycine allele) has been associated with a more positive response to atypical anti-psychotic medication (Szekeres et al., 2004).

Four antipsychotic medications have moderate to high affinity to the DRD3 receptor. Affinity refers to the ability of a drug to bind to a receptor. Haloperidol is a typical antipsychotic that has the highest affinity (Table 16.2).

Olanzapine

An interaction between rs6280 (i.e., Ser9Gly) and the promoter variant −205A/G has been reported that predicts improvement in the positive

TABLE 16.2. Antipsychotic drug affinity for DRD3 receptors in nM

Antipsychotic Drugs	DRD3 Receptor Affinity (nM)
Haloperidol	High (2.5)
Ziprasidone	Moderate (7.2)
Aripiprazole	Moderate (9.1)
Risperidone	Moderate (9.6)
Olanzapine	Low (50)
Clozapine	Low (240)
Quetiapine	Low (940)

Duncan et al. (1999); and Lawler et al. (1999).

symptoms of schizophrenia. Subjects with schizophrenia who had the thymine allele (i.e., the glycine allele) of rs6280 and the glycine allele of –205A/G were most likely to have an improvement in their positive symptoms when treated with olanzapine (Staddon et al., 2002).

Risperidone

A study of Korean patients with schizophrenia who were treated with risperidone reported that those patients who were homozygous for the thymine allele (i.e., the glycine allele) of rs6280 (i.e., Ser9Gly) had better symptom relief than did patients who would have had one or two copies of the cytosine allele (i.e., the serine allele). Those patients who had one or more copies of the cytosine allele (i.e., the serine allele) and who were also homozygous for the cytosine allele of rs6313 (i.e., 102T/C) of the HTR2A gene were the least likely to respond to risperidone (Kim et al., 2008).

ADVERSE EFFECTS OF ANTIPSYCHOTICS

Tardive Dyskinesia and Extrapyramidal Side Effects

The thymine allele (i.e., the glycine allele) of rs6280 has been reported to have a higher dopamine activity and has been associated with an increased risk of developing tardive dyskinesia (Arranz & de Leon, 2007).

Patients who were homozygous for the thymine allele of rs6280 were more likely to develop drug-induced tardive dyskinesia (Steen et al., 1997). This homozygous thymine genotype was also more common in patients with akathisia (Eichhammer et al., 2000). In yet another positive report, the homozygous thymine genotype of rs6280 was reported to be associated with a greater risk of tardive dyskinesia when compared to patients who were either heterozygous for the glycine and cytosine alleles or homozygous for the cytosine alleles. The mean Abnormal Involuntary Movement Score (AIMS) was 14.2 for the homozygous thymine genotype, as compared to 3.9 for the heterozygous thymine and cytosine genotype and 3.5 for the cytosine homozygous genotype (Basile et al., 1999).

Other studies have further supported the finding that the thymine allele of rs6280 is more frequently associated with tardive dyskinesia (de Leon et al., 2005; Liao et al., 2001; Segman et al., 1999). While this association with tardive dyskinesia has not been universally found (Chong et al., 2003; Lovlie et al., 2000), a meta-analysis has confirmed that the thymine allele (i.e., the glycine allele) of rs6280 is associated with increased risk of tardive dyskinesia (Bakker et al., 2006).

In a Chinese sample of patients with schizophrenia, the rs6280 heterozygotic patients were at some increased risk for tardive dyskinesia. However, the presence of the thymine allele (i.e., the glycine allele) of rs6280 in combination with the valine allele of the manganese superoxide dismutase gene (MnSOD) was more significantly associated with tardive dyskinesia (Zhang et al., 2003). The MnSOD gene is associated with mitochondrial free-radical scavenging, and the valine allele of this gene is associated with either less protection against oxidative stress or more mitochondrial damage.

A Canadian sample of patients with schizophrenia who were homozygous for the thymine allele (i.e., the glycine allele) of rs6280 also had higher scores on the AIMS. When these subjects were treated with haloperidol, the metabolism in their caudate and putamen was increased, as compared to subjects who had one or two copies of the cytosine allele (i.e., the serine allele) and who did not demonstrate an increase in metabolism in these regions (Potkin et al., 2002).

CLINICAL IMPLICATIONS

The primary use of DRD3 genotyping has been to provide guidance on the selection of antipsychotic medications.

Clinical Case 15

A 31-year-old Italian woman who was a violinist in a prestigious symphony orchestra was diagnosed with bipolar disorder and experienced intense delusions of grandeur. Her mother had been treated for 29 years for schizophrenia and, for much of this time, she was prescribed haloperidol. The mother of the patient did develop tardive dyskinesia, but this condition improved after her haloperidol was discontinued. The mother was subsequently treated effectively with olanzapine. The violinist's psychiatrist hoped that treatment with an atypical antipsychotic medication would be less likely to result in the development of extrapyramidal side effects. Furthermore, he reasoned that olanzapine might be a good choice for this patient, given that her mother had responded to olanzapine. However, prior to selecting an antipsychotic medication, her psychiatrist ordered pharmacogenomic testing (Table 16.3).

TABLE 16.3. Pharmacogenomic report of case 15

Pharmacogenomic Report of Case 15			
Gene	Gene Variant	Genotype	Clinical Implication
CYP2D6	N/A	*3/*10	Poor CYP2D6 metabolizer
CYP2C19	N/A	*2/*2	Poor CYP2C19 metabolizer
CYP2C9	N/A	*1/*1	Extensive CYP2C9 metabolizer
CYP1A2	N/A	*1A/*1F	Extensive CYP1A2 metabolizer
COMT	rs4680	G/G	High Activity
HTR2A	rs6311	G/G	Worse response to antipsychotic medication
HTR2A	rs6313	T/C	Worse response to antipsychotic medication
HTR2C	rs3813929	C/C	Greater risk of weight gain
DRD3	rs6280	T/T	Greater risk of tardive dyskinesia

On review of the pharmacogenomic report, the psychiatrist realized that, based on her HTR2A, HTR2C, and DRD3 genotypes, his patient was at high risk of having a poor therapeutic response to an atypical antipsychotic medication, as well as having an increased risk for developing side effects. Additionally, the report suggested that, based on her CYP2D6 and CYP2C19 genotypes, his patient might well have difficulty metabolizing most atypical antipsychotic medications. Consequently, her psychiatrist decided not to prescribe olanzapine, but instead initiated treatment with valproic acid.

KEY CLINICAL CONSIDERATIONS

- The thymine allele of rs6280 (i.e., Ser9Gly) has been associated with a more positive response to atypical antipsychotic medications. However, this allele has also been associated with the development of tardive dyskinesia.
- Continued research is needed to clarify the potential risks and benefits of DRD3 genotypic variations and treatment with antipsychotic medications.

REFERENCES

Adams, D. H., Close, S., Farmen, M., Downing, A. M., Breier, A., & Houston, J. P. (2008). Dopamine receptor D3 genotype association with greater acute positive symptom remission with olanzapine therapy in predominately Caucasian patients with chronic schizophrenia or schizoaffective disorder. *Human Psychopharmacology, 23*(4), 267–274.

Arranz, M. J., & de Leon, J. (2007). Pharmacogenetics and pharmacogenomics of schizophrenia: a review of last decade of research. *Molecular Psychiatry, 12*(8), 707–747.

Bakker, P. R., van Harten, P. N., & van Os, J. (2006). Antipsychotic-induced tardive dyskinesia and the Ser9Gly polymorphism in the DRD3 gene: a meta analysis. *Schizophrenia Research, 83*(2–3), 185–192.

Basile, V. S., Masellis, M., Badri, F., Paterson A. D., Meltzer, H. Y., Liberbman, J. A., et al. (1999). Association of the MscI polymorphism of the dopamine D3 receptor gene with tardive dyskinesia in schizophrenia. *Neuropsychopharmacology, 21*(1), 17–27.

Chong, S. A., Tan, E. C., Tan, C. H., Mythily, & Chan, Y. H. (2003). Polymorphisms of dopamine receptors and tardive dyskinesia among Chinese patients with schizophrenia. *American Journal of Medical Genetics Part B, Neuropsychiatric Genetics, 116B*(1), 51–54.

de Leon, J., Susce, M. T., Pan, R. M., Koch, W. H., & Wedlund, P. J. (2005). Polymorphic variations in GSTM1, GSTT1, PgP, CYP2D6, CYP3A5, and dopamine D2 and D3 receptors and their association with tardive dyskinesia in severe mental illness. *Journal of Clinical Psychopharmacology, 25*(5), 448–456.

Duncan, G. E., Zorn, S., & Lieberman, J. A. (1999). Mechanisms of typical and atypical antipsychotic drug action in relation to dopamine and NMDA receptor hypofunction hypotheses of schizophrenia. *Molecular Psychiatry, 4*(5), 418–428.

Eichhammer, P., Albus, M., Borrmann-Hassenbach, M., Schoeler, A., Putzhammer, A., Frick, U., et al. (2000). Association of dopamine D3-receptor gene variants with neuroleptic induced akathisia in schizophrenic patients: a generalization of Steen's study on DRD3 and tardive dyskinesia. *American Journal of Medical Genetics, 96*(2), 187–191.

Joyce, J. N. (2001). Dopamine D3 receptor as a therapeutic target for antipsychotic and antiparkinsonian drugs. *Pharmacology & Therapeutics, 90*(2–3), 231-259.

Kim, B., Choi, E. Y., Kim, C. Y., Song, K., & Joo, Y. H. (2008). Could HTR2A T102C and DRD3 Ser9Gly predict clinical improvement in patients with acutely exacerbated schizophrenia? Results from treatment responses to risperidone in a naturalistic setting. *Human Psychopharmacology, 23*(1), 61–67.

Lawler, C. P., Prioleau, C., Lewis, M. M., Mak, C., Jiang, D., Schetz, J.A., et al. (1999). Interactions of the novel antipsychotic aripiprazole (OPC-14597) with dopamine and serotonin receptor subtypes. *Neuropsychopharmacology, 20*(6), 612–627.

Liao, D. L., Yeh, Y. C., Chen, H. M., Chen, H., Hong, C. J., & Tsai, S. J. (2001). Association between the Ser9Gly polymorphism of the dopamine D3 receptor gene and tardive dyskinesia in Chinese schizophrenic patients. *Neuropsychobiology, 44*(2), 95–98.

Lovlie, R., Daly, A. K., Blennerhassett, R., Ferrier, N., & Steen, V. M. (2000). Homozygosity for the Gly-9 variant of the dopamine D3 receptor and risk for tardive dyskinesia in schizophrenic patients. *International Journal of Neuropsychopharmacology, 3*(1), 61–65.

Ma, G., He, Z., Fang, W., Tang, W., Huang, K., Li, Z., et al. (2008). The Ser9Gly polymorphism of the dopamine D3 receptor gene and risk of schizophrenia: an association study and a large meta-analysis. *Schizophrenia Research, 101*(1–3), 26–35.

Martinez-Marignac, V. L., & Bianchi, N. O. (2006). Prevalence of dopamine and 5HT2C receptor polymorphisms in Amerindians and in an urban population from Argentina. *American Journal of Human Biology, 18*(6), 822–828.

Potkin, S. G., Kennedy, J. L., & Basile, V. S. (2002). Brain imaging and pharmacogenetics in Alzheimer's disease and schizophrenia. In B. Lerer (Ed.), *Pharmacogenetics of Psychotropic Drugs* (pp. 439). Jerusalem: Cambridge University Press.

Scharfetter, J. (2004). Pharmacogenetics of dopamine receptors and response to antipsychotic drugs in schizophrenia—an update. *Pharmacogenomics, 5*(6), 691–698.

Segman, R., Neeman, T., Heresco-Levy, U., Finkel, B., Karagichev, L., Schlafman, M., Dorevitch, A., et al. (1999). Genotypic association between the dopamine D3 receptor and tardive dyskinesia in chronic schizophrenia. *Molecular Psychiatry, 4*(3), 247–253.

Staddon, S., Arranz, M. J., Mancama, D., Mata, I., & Kerwin, R. W. (2002). Clinical applications of pharmacogenetics in psychiatry. *Psychopharmacology, 162*(1), 18–23.

Steen, V. M., Lovlie, R., MacEwan, T., & McCreadie, R. G. (1997). Dopamine D3-receptor gene variant and susceptibility to tardive dyskinesia in schizophrenic patients. *Molecular Psychiatry, 2*(2), 139–145.

Szekeres, G., Keri, S., Juhasz, A., Rimanoczy, A., Szendi, I., Czimmer, C., & Janka, Z. (2004). Role of dopamine D3 receptor (DRD3) and dopamine transporter (DAT) polymorphism in cognitive dysfunctions and therapeutic response to atypical antipsychotics in patients with schizophrenia. *American Journal of Medical Genetics. Part B, Neuropsychiatric Genetics: The Official Publication of the International Society of Psychiatric Genetics, 124B*(1), 1–5.

Xuan, J., Zhao, X., He, G., Yu, L., Wang, L., Tang, W., et al. (2008). Effects of the dopamine D3 receptor (DRD3) gene polymorphisms on risperidone response: a pharmacogenetic study. *Neuropsychopharmacology, 33*(2), 305–311.

Zhang, Z. J., Zhang, X. B., Hou, G., Yao, H., & Reynolds, G. P. (2003). Interaction between polymorphisms of the dopamine D3 receptor and manganese superoxide dismutase genes in susceptibility to tardive dyskinesia. *Psychiatric Genetics, 13*(3), 187–192.

17

THE DOPAMINE D4 RECEPTOR GENE

The dopamine receptor gene (DRD4) encodes for the D4 subtype of the dopamine receptor. The D4 subtype is relatively homologous to both the D2 and D3 subtypes of the dopamine receptors. All three of these subtypes are G-protein coupled receptors that inhibit the enzyme adenylyl cyclase. The D4 subtype is located predominantly in the prefrontal cortex.

The density of the D4 receptors has been reported to be greater in the brains of patients with schizophrenia (Lung et al., 2002; Seeman et al., 1993a; Van Tol et al., 1991). Conversely, the density of D4 receptors has been reported to be lower in the brains of patients with Parkinson disease (Seeman et al., 1993b). The D4 receptor is thus a target for many drugs that have been used to treat patients with schizophrenia and Parkinson disease.

Mutations in the DRD4 gene have been associated with multiple behavioral phenotypes. These include attention-deficit hyperactivity disorder (ADHD) (Brookes et al., 2006), and the personality trait of novelty seeking (Ebstein et al., 1996; Munafo et al., 2008; Okuyama et al., 2000).

LOCATION AND GENE VARIATION

DRD4 is located on chromosome 11. The specific location of the gene is on the short arm of chromosome 11 at 11p15.5 (Fig. 17.1).

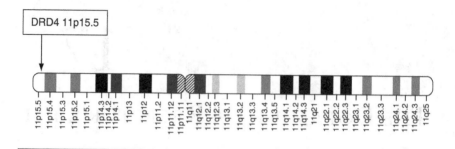

FIGURE 17.1. Chromosome 11 with arrow to designate the location of the DRD4.

DRD4 consists of 3,399 nucleotides or 3.4 kilobases and contains four exons, which are composed of 1,360 nucleotides. These exons code for a polypeptide that is composed of 419 amino acids (Fig. 17.2).

Table 17.1 provides a list of the most well-studied DRD4 alleles and includes both the ancestral and mutant nucleotides. Each allele is described in the following technical discussion.

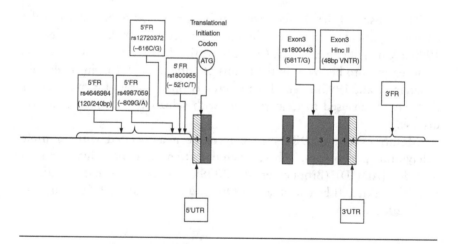

FIGURE 17.2. DRD4 structure illustrating the location of the four exons and the single nucleotide polymorphisms that define the most important DRD4 alleles. Wang et al. (2004).

Table 17.1. The locations of nucleotide changes that define the most well-studied DRD4 alleles

refSNP ID & Aliases	Nucleotide Location	Ancestral Allele	Mutant Variant
rs4646984 or 120(short)/240(long)	5' FR	120	240
rs4987059 or -809G/A	−809	G	A
rs12720372 or -616C/G or AVAII	−616	C	G
rs1800955 or -521C/T or BssHII or FspI	−521	C	T
rs1800443 or 581T/G or Val194Gly	581	T	G
HincII or 48 bp VNTR	Exon 3	4-repeat	7-repeat

Technical Discussion of DRD4 Variations

Each of the most-well studied DRD4 alleles is described in this technical discussion.

rs4646984 or the 120 (Short Allele)/240 (Long Allele) bp Repeat Variation

rs4646984 is located about 1.24-kb upstream of the translational initiation codon. Its location is also upstream of the promoter region. The long form, which is sometimes referred to as the 120 duplication allele, contains 240 bp. The short form contains 120 base pairs. The long allele has been reported to have lower transcriptional activity than the short form (D'Souza et al., 2004).

rs4987059 or –809G/A

rs4987059 is the result of a guanine to adenine change at nucleotide location −809 in the promoter region.

rs12720372 or –616C/G or AVAII

rs12720372 is the result of a cytosine to guanine change at nucleotide location −616 in the promoter region. This polymorphism has also been identified using the restriction fragment enzyme, AVAII (Barr et al., 2001; Lowe et al., 2004; Okuyama et al., 2000).

rs1800955 or –521C/T or BssHII or FspI

rs1800955 is the result of a cytosine to thymine change at nucleotide location –521 in the promoter region. This polymorphism has also been identified using two different restriction fragment enzymes, BssHII and FspI. The thymine allele has been reported to have 40% less transcription efficiency when compared to the cytosine allele (Barr et al., 2001; Okuyama, 2000). Furthermore, the thymine allele has been associated with the personality trait of novelty seeking (Munafo et al., 2008).

(Continued)

rs1800443 or 581T/G or Val194Gly

rs1800443 is the result of a thymine to guanine change at nucleotide location 581 in exon 3. This results in an amino acid change from a valine to a glycine at amino acid position 194. The guanine allele (i.e., glycine allele) has only been identified in samples of African origin (Seeman et al., 1994). The guanine allele decreases the sensitivity of the DRD4 receptor to dopamine, as well as to clozapine and olanzapine (Liu et al., 1996).

HincII or 48 bp Variable Number Tandem Repeats (VNTR) in Exon 3

HincII is located in exon 3 and is defined by the number of 16 amino acid repeated sequences present (Cohen et al., 1999). The amino acids coded by these repeated sequences of 48 nucleotides are located in the third cytoplasmic loop of the D4 receptor (Van Tol et al., 1992). Alleles have been reported (D'Souza et al., 2004) that contain between two and eleven repeated 48-bp sequences. The polymorphisms created by these multiple repeats produce proteins that contain polypeptides in the cytoplasmic loop that range from 32 to 176 amino acids in length. The cytoplasmic loop of the DRD4 receptor is thought to bind G-proteins that link receptor activation to the creation of intracellular second-messengers (Cohen et al., 1999).

The 7-repeat allele of the 48-bp variable-number tandem repeat (VNTR) has been referred to as the "long allele" and has been reported to be less responsive to dopamine stimulation than some of the shorter versions of this allele. The 7-repeat allele of this 48-bp VNTR has also been associated with novelty seeking, as has the thymine allele of rs1800955 (i.e., –521C/T) (Ebstein et al., 1996).

The 4-repeat allele of the 48-bp VNTR has been found in virtually all populations and is considered to be the ancestral allele (Chang et al., 1996; Ding et al, 2002). However, the evolution of the 2-repeat allele and the 7-repeat allele is believed to have occurred before the global dispersion out of Africa, since these newer alleles are commonly found in widely diverse geographical locations (Wang et al., 2004).

GENOTYPIC VARIANCE ACROSS GEOGRAPHIC ANCESTRY

HincII or the 48-bp VNTR in Exon 3

Most of the reports on allele frequencies of different groups of patients based on geographical ancestry have focused on the 48-bp VNTR in exon 3. Although the 4-repeat ancestral allele is the most common in almost all populations, the 7-repeat allele is quite common in North American populations, ranging from 20% to 40%. The 7-repeat allele is less common in many Asian populations, and it does not occur at all in the Han Chinese (Chang et al., 1996).

In a North American sample composed of only individuals of European ancestry, normal control subjects had a 4-repeat allele frequency of 61% and a 7-repeat allele frequency of 26% (Cohen et al., 1999). In contrast to the controls in this study, subjects with schizophrenia who were taking typical antipsychotic medications had a 4-repeat allele frequency of 83% and a 7-repeat allele frequency of 9%.

A Han Chinese sample of children with attention-deficit hyperactivity disorder (ADHD) was found to have a 2-repeat allele frequency of 33% (Leung et al., 2005). However, in another study of Han Chinese, the 2-repeat allele frequency was only 0.6%. In this second report, the most common allele was the 5-repeat, which had an allele frequency of 71% (Zhao et al., 2005). In a sample of Taiwanese subjects, the 4-repeat allele was the most common, with an allele frequency of 73% (Hwu et al., 1998).

Considerable variability of the 4-repeat and 7-repeat alleles has been reported in South American samples (Martinez-Marignac & Bianchi, 2006). Similarly, in a sample of Pakistani subjects, considerable variability exists between subjects from the north of the country versus subjects from the south. However, throughout Pakistan, the 4-repeat allele was the most common, ranging from 70% to 83% (Mansoor et al., 2008).

rs1800443 or 581T/G

The guanine variant of rs1800443 (i.e., 581T/G) has not been found in samples of European ancestry (Seeman et al., 1994). However, the guanine variant was documented to have occurred in 13% of an Afro-Caribbean sample.

rs12720372 or –616C/G

The rs12720372 (i.e., –616C/G) allele frequency has been reported for a Han Chinese sample (Xing et al., 2003). The cytosine allele had an allele frequency of 37%, whereas the thymine allele had an allele frequency of 63%.

rs1800955 or –521C/T

In a Han Chinese sample, the cytosine allele of rs1800955 (i.e., –521C/T) had an allele frequency of 42%, whereas the thymine allele had an allele frequency of 58% (Xing et al., 2003).

ANTIDEPRESSANT MEDICATIONS

No consistent research findings have linked variability in DRD4 with antidepressant therapeutic response or side effects.

ANTIPSYCHOTIC MEDICATIONS

Considerable variations in the affinities of antipsychotic medications to the DRD4 receptor have been reported (Seeman & Van Tol, 1994) (Table 17.2). Furthermore, some variants of DRD4, such as the guanine allele (i.e., the glycine allele) of rs1800443 (i.e., 581T/G or Val194Gly), have a particularly low affinity to clozapine (Liu et al., 1996).

TABLE 17.2. Antipsychotic drug affinity for DRD4 receptors in nM

Antipsychotic Drugs	D4 Receptor Affinity (nM)
Haloperidol	High (3.3)
Risperidone	Moderate (8.5)
Ziprasidone	Low (32)
Clozapine	Low (47)
Olanzapine	Low (50)
Aripiprazole	Low (260)
Quetiapine	Low (2200)

Van Tol et al. (1991); Duncan et al. (1999) and Lawler et al. (1999).

Typical Antipsychotic Medications

A differential response to the typical antipsychotic medications has been reported to occur in subjects who have different variants of the 48-bp VNTR in the third exon. Specifically, a study of North American patients of European ancestry who had the 7-repeat allele were less likely to respond to typical antipsychotic medication than were subjects with shorter forms of the allele, such as the 4-repeat allele (Cohen et al., 1999).

A similar relationship was demonstrated in a sample of patients in Taiwan who had schizophrenia. Those patients who were homozygous for the 4-repeat allele of the 48-bp repeat in the third exon were more likely to respond to typical antipsychotic medication than were subjects with copies of the 2-repeat allele. No patients in this study had a copy of the 7-repeat allele (Hwu et al., 1998).

Clozapine

Clozapine has a higher affinity to the D4 receptor than either the D2 receptor or the D3 receptor (Van Tol et al., 1991). In a sample composed primarily of subjects of European ancestry, responders to clozapine were more likely to have the 7-repeat allele of the 48-bp VNTR in the third exon than did patients who had responded to typical antipsychotic medications (Cohen et al., 1999).

In a sample of Han Chinese, responders to clozapine were more likely to be homozygous for the 5-repeat allele. No subject in this study had the 7-repeat allele (Zhao et al., 2005).

ADVERSE EFFECTS OF ANTIPSYCHOTICS

Tardive Dyskinesia and Extrapyramidal Side Effects

The 120-bp duplication and the thymine allele of rs1800955 (i.e., –521C/T) are two polymorphisms of DRD4 that define a haplotype that has been shown to be associated with an increased risk for tardive dyskinesia in an Indian sample (Srivastava et al., 2006).

Variation in the 48-bp VNTR in the third exon has also been associated with tardive dyskinesia. Specifically, in an Italian sample of patients with schizophrenia, no subjects who were homozygous for the long allele of the 48-bp VNTR polymorphism developed tardive dyskinesia, whereas 80% of the subjects who were homozygous for the short allele of the 48-bp VNTR did develop tardive dyskinesia (Lattuada et al., 2004).

METHYLPHENIDATE

Methylphenidate has been reported to be effective in approximately 70% of patients with ADHD (Seeger et al., 2001). Less effective symptom response to methylphenidate has been associated with having one or more copies of the longer 7-repeat allele. The response rate of patients with a copy of the 7-repeat allele of the 48-bp VNTR in the third exon of DRD4 has been reported to be only 58%, whereas patients without the 7-repeat allele have been reported to have as high as a 95% response rate (Hamarman et al., 2004).

In a similar, but independent study, preschool subjects with ADHD who had a 7-repeat allele required higher doses of methylphenidate to achieve a comparable symptom response (McGough et al., 2006). Increasing the dose of methylphenidate in three children with the 7-repeat allele was, however, associated with social withdrawal.

A study of Korean children with ADHD reported that those who were homozygous for the 4-repeat allele of the 48-bp VNTR in the third exon had the best response to methylphenidate (Cheon et al., 2007). Although good response in children without the 7-repeat allele has been a relatively consistent finding, not all studies have reported this association. In a recent small study of Hungarian children, subjects without a 7-repeat allele did not do significantly better than other genotypes (Kereszturi et al., 2008).

An interaction between the 48-bp VNTR in the third exon of DRD4 and rs4495541 of SLC6A4 has been reported to be associated in treatment with methylphenidate. Specifically, patients with a 7-repeat allele of the 48-bp by VNTR in the third exon who also were homozygous for the long form of the indel promoter polymorphism of SLC6A4 were less likely to respond to methylphenidate. These individuals also had higher prolactin levels (Seeger et al., 2001).

TRANSDERMAL NICOTINE PATCH

An association has been reported between variation in the 48-bp VNTR polymorphism in the third exon of DRD4 and response to transdermal nicotine patch treatment of nicotine dependence (David et al., 2008). Specifically, having one or more copies of the long allele, defined as the 7-repeat allele, was associated with having a higher rate of abstinence from smoking at 12-week follow-up. A possible mechanism of action for this association is that the 7-repeat allele is believed to code for DRD4 receptors with a lower dopaminergic tone in the mesocortico-limbic region than would be produced in individuals with shorter variants.

CLINICAL IMPLICATIONS

Clinical pharmacogenomic testing currently includes the documentation of the genotype of the 48-bp polymorphism of the third exon of DRD4, in conjunction with the indel promoter polymorphism of SLC6A4. Using just these two genotypes, it is possible to identify patients with ADHD who are more likely to do well with methylphenidate treatment. By additionally genotyping CYP2D6, patients who may have atypical responses to amphetamine salts and atomoxetine can also be identified.

Clinical Case 16

A 10-year-old boy underwent a clinical evaluation for behavior problems in school and difficulty completing homework assignments. His parents were both physicians and they believed that their son was a gifted child who was primarily having difficulty concentrating at school. The clinical evaluation revealed that their son did have sufficient attentional and hyperactive symptomatology to meet the diagnostic criteria for ADHD. His parents requested that a pharmacogenomic panel be genotyped for their son in order to provide evidence-based guidance in the selection of an appropriate medication (Table 17.3).

TABLE 17.3. Pharmacogenomic report of case 16

Gene	Gene Variant	Genotype	Clinical Implication
		Pharmacogenomic Report of Case 16	
CYP2D6	N/A	*1/*2ADup	Ultra-rapid CYP2D6 metabolizer
CYP2C19	N/A	*1/*2	Intermediate CYP2C19 metabolizer
CYP2C9	N/A	*1/*3	Intermediate CYP2C9 metabolizer
CYP1A2	N/A	*1A/*1F	Extensive CYP1A2 metabolizer
COMT	rs4680	G/G	High Activity
SLC6A4	rs4495541	Short/Short	Positive interaction with homozygous 4-repeat VNTR of DRD4
DRD4	VNTR in exon 3	4-repeat/4-repeat	Positive response to methylphenidate

Genotyping revealed that the patient was homozygous for the 4-repeat allele of the 48-bp VNTR in the third exon of DRD4 and homozygous for the short form of the indel promoter polymorphism of SLC6A4. This combination of predictive genotypes would indicate that he has a relatively high probability of responding to methylphenidate. Additionally, given his ultra-rapid 2D6 metabolizer phenotype, he would be unlikely to achieve an adequate serum level of amphetamine compounds or atomoxetine at recommended dosages.

Clinical Case 17

An 8-year-old girl of European ancestry underwent a clinical evaluation for distractibility and poor performance at school. The evaluation revealed that she clearly met the diagnostic criteria for ADHD. Given that her parents felt strongly that she could benefit from medication, pharmacogenomic testing was ordered (Table 17.4).

(*Continued*)

TABLE 17.4. Pharmacogenomic report of case 17

		Pharmacogenomic Report of Case 17	
Gene	Gene Variant	Genotype	Clinical Implication
CYP2D6	N/A	*1/*2A	Extensive CYP2D6 metabolizer
CYP2C19	N/A	*1/*8	Intermediate CYP2C19 metabolizer
CYP2C9	N/A	*1/*1	Extensive CYP2C9 metabolizer
CYP1A2	N/A	*1F/*1F	Extensive CYP1A2 metabolizer
COMT	rs4680	G/G	High Activity
SLC6A4	rs4495541	Long/ Long	Less likely to respond to methylphenidate when this genotype occurs with the homozygous 7 repeat allele of the 48 bp VNTR in the third exon of DRD4
DRD4	VNTR in exon 3	7-repeat/ 7-repeat	Less likely to respond to methylphenidate

Genotyping revealed that the patient was homozygous for the 7-repeat allele of the 48-bp VNTR in the third exon of DRD4 and homozygous for the long form of the indel promoter polymorphism of SLC6A4. Given these two genotypes, she would have a relatively low probability of responding to methylphenidate. However, given her extensive 2D6 metabolizer phenotype, she would be able to tolerate recommended doses of amphetamine compounds and atomoxetine.

KEY CLINICAL CONSIDERATION

- Patients with ADHD are more likely to respond positively to methylphenidate if they are homozygous for the 4-repeat allele of the VNTR in exon 3 of DRD4.

REFERENCES

Barr, C. L., Feng, Y., Wigg, K. G., Schachar, R., Tannock, R., Roberts, W., et al. (2001). 5'-untranslated region of the dopamine D$_4$ receptor gene and attention-deficit hyperactivity disorder. *American Journal of Medical Genetics, 105*(1), 84–90.

Brookes, K., Xu, X., Chen, W., Zhou, K., Neale, B., Lowe, N., et al. (2006). The analysis of 51 genes in DSM-IV combined type attention deficit hyperactivity disorder: association signals in DRD4, DAT1 and 16 other genes. *Molecular Psychiatry, 11*(10), 934–953.

Chang, F. M., Kidd, J. R., Livak, K. J., Pakstis, A. J., & Kidd, K. K. (1996). The world-wide distribution of allele frequencies at the human dopamine D_4 receptor locus. *Human Genetics, 98*(1), 91–101.

Cheon, K.-A., Kim, B.-N., & Cho, S.-C. (2007). Association of 4-repeat allele of the dopamine D_4 receptor gene exon III polymorphism and response to methylphenidate treatment in Korean ADHD children. *Neuropsychopharmacology, 32*(6), 1377–1383.

Cohen, B. M., Ennulat, D. J., Centorrino, F., Matthysse, S., Konieczna, H., Chu, H. M., & Cherkerzian, S. (1999). Polymorphisms of the dopamine D_4 receptor and response to antipsychotic drugs. *Psychopharmacology, 141*(1), 6–10.

D'Souza, U., Russa, C., Tahira, E., Milla, J., McGuffina, P., Ashersona, P., & Craiga, I. (2004). Functional effects of a tandem duplication polymorphism in the 5' flanking region of the DRD4 gene. *Biological Psychiatry, 56*(9), 691–697.

David, S. P., Munafo, M. R., Murphy, M. F., Proctor, M., Walton, R. T., & Johnstone, E. C. (2008). Genetic variation in the dopamine D_4 receptor (DRD4) gene and smoking cessation: follow-up of a randomised clinical trial of transdermal nicotine patch. *The Pharmacogenomics Journal, 8*(2), 122–128.

Ding, Y. (2002). Evidence of positive selection acting at the human dopamine receptor D_4 gene locus. *Proceedings of the National Academy of Sciences of the United States of America, 99*(1), 309–314.

Duncan, G. E., Zorn, S., & Lieberman, J. A. (1999). Mechanisms of typical and atypical antipsychotic drug action in relation to dopamine and NMDA receptor hypofunction hypotheses of schizophrenia. *Molecular Psychiatry, 4*(5), 418–428.

Ebstein, R. P., Novick, O., Umansky, R., Priel, B., Osher, Y., Blaine, D., et al. (1996). Dopamine D_4 receptor (D4DR) exon III polymorphism associated with the human personality trait of Novelty Seeking. *Nature Genetics, 12*(1), 78–80.

Hamarman, S., Fossella, J., Ulger, C., Brimacombe, M., & Dermody, J. (2004). Dopamine receptor 4 (DRD4) 7-repeat allele predicts methylphenidate dose response in children with attention deficit hyperactivity disorder: a pharmacogenetic study. *Journal of Child & Adolescent Psychopharmacology, 14*(4), 564–574.

Hwu, H. G., Hong, C. J., Lee, Y. L., Lee, P. C., & Lee, S. F. (1998). Dopamine D_4 receptor gene polymorphisms and neuroleptic response in schizophrenia. *Biological Psychiatry, 44*(6), 483–487.

Kereszturi, E., Tarnok, Z., Bognar, E., Lakatos, K., Farkas, L., Gadoros, J., et al. (2008). Catechol-O-methyltransferase Val158Met polymorphism is associated with methylphenidate response in ADHD children. *American Journal of Medical Genetics Part B: Neuropsychiatric Genetics, 147B*(8), 1431–1435.

Lattuada, E., Cavallaro, R., Serretti, A., Lorenzi, C., & Smeraldi, E. (2004). Tardive dyskinesia and DRD2, DRD3, DRD4, 5-HT2A variants in schizophrenia: an association study with repeated assessment. *International Journal of Neuropsychopharmacology, 7*(4), 489–493.

Lawler, C. P., Prioleau, C., Lewis, M. M., Mak, C., Jiang, D., Schetz, J. A., et al. (1999). Interactions of the novel antipsychotic aripiprazole (OPC-14597) with dopamine and serotonin receptor subtypes. *Neuropsychopharmacology, 20*(6), 612–627.

Leung, P. W., Lee, C. C., Hung, S. F., Ho, T. P., Tang, C. P., Kwong, S. L., et al. (2005). Dopamine receptor D_4 (DRD4) gene in Han Chinese children with attention-deficit/hyperactivity disorder (ADHD): increased prevalence of the 2-repeat allele. *American Journal of Medical Genetics. Part B, Neuropsychiatric Genetics : The Official Publication of the International Society of Psychiatric Genetics, 133B*(1), 54–56.

Liu, I. S., Seeman, P., Sanyal, S., Ulpian, C., Rodgers-Johnson, P. E., Serjeant, G. R., & Van Tol, H. H. (1996). Dopamine D_4 receptor variant in Africans, D_4valine194glycine, is insensitive to dopamine and clozapine: report of a homozygous individual. *American Journal of Medical Genetics, 61*(3), 277–282.

Lowe, N., Kirley, A., Mullins, C., Fitzgerald, M., Gill, M., & Hawi, Z. (2004). Multiple marker analysis at the promoter region of the DRD4 gene and ADHD: evidence of linkage and association with the SNP -616. *American Journal of Medical Genetics, Part B, Neuropsychiatric Genetics, 131*(1), 33–37.

Lung, F.-W., Tzeng, D.-S., & Shu, B.-C. (2002). Ethnic heterogeneity in allele variation in the DRD4 gene in schizophrenia. *Schizophrenia Research, 57*(2–3), 239–245.

Mansoor, A., Mazhar, K., & Qamar, R. (2008). VNTR polymorphism of the DRD4 locus in different Pakistani ethnic groups. *Genetic Testing, 12*(2), 299–304.

Martinez-Marignac, V. L., & Bianchi, N. O. (2006). Prevalence of dopamine and 5HT2C receptor polymorphisms in Amerindians and in an urban population from Argentina. *American Journal of Human Biology, 18*(6), 822–828.

McGough, J., McCracken, J., Swanson, J., Riddle, M., Kollins, S., Greenhill, L., et al. (2006). Pharmacogenetics of methylphenidate response in preschoolers with ADHD. [comment]. *Journal of the American Academy of Child & Adolescent Psychiatry, 45*(11), 1314–1322.

Munafo, M. R., Yalcin, B., Willis-Owen, S. A., & Flint, J. (2008). Association of the dopamine D_4 receptor (DRD4) gene and approach-related personality traits: meta-analysis and new data. *Biological Psychiatry, 63*(2), 197–206.

Okuyama, Y., Ishiguro, H., Nankai, M., Shibuya, H., Watanabe, A., & Arinami, T. (2000). Identification of a polymorphism in the promoter region of DRD4 associated with the human novelty seeking personality trait. *Molecular Psychiatry, 5*(1), 64–69.

Seeger, G., Schloss, P., & Schmidt, M. H. (2001). Marker gene polymorphisms in hyperkinetic disorder—predictors of clinical response to treatment with methylphenidate? *Neuroscience Letters 313*(1–2), 45–48.

Seeman, P., Guan, H. C., & Van Tol, H. H. (1993a). Dopamine D_4 receptors elevated in schizophrenia. *Nature, 365*(6445), 441–445.

Seeman, P., Guan, H. C., Van Tol, H. H., & Niznik, H. B. (1993b). Low density of dopamine D_4 receptors in Parkinson's, schizophrenia, and control brain striata. *Synapse, 14*(4), 247–253.

Seeman, P., Ulpian, C., Chouinard, G., Van Tol, H. H., Dwosh, H., Lieberman, J. A., et al. (1994). Dopamine D_4 receptor variant, D_4GLYCINE194, in Africans, but not in Caucasians: no association with schizophrenia. *American Journal of Medical Genetics, 54*(4), 384–390.

Seeman, P., & Van Tol, H. H. (1994). Dopamine receptor pharmacology. *Trends in Pharmacological Sciences, 15*(7), 264–270.

Srivastava, V., Varma, P. G., Prasad, S., Semwal, P., Nimgaonkar, V. L., Lerer, B., et al. (2006). Genetic susceptibility to tardive dyskinesia among schizophrenia subjects: IV. Role of dopaminergic pathway gene polymorphisms. *Pharmacogenetics & Genomics, 16*(2), 111–117.

Van Tol, H. H., Wu, C. M., Guan, H. C., Ohara, K., Bunzow, J. R., Civelli, O., et al. (1992). Multiple dopamine D_4 receptor variants in the human population. *Nature, 358*(6382), 149–152.

Van Tol, H. H., Bunzow, J. R., Guan, H. C., Sunahara, R. K., Seeman, P., Niznik, H. B., et al. (1991). Cloning of the gene for a human dopamine D_4 receptor with high affinity for the antipsychotic clozapine. *Nature, 350*(6319), 610–614.

Wang, E., Ding, Y., Flodman, P., Kidd, J., Kidd, K., Grady, D., et al. (2004). The genetic architecture of selection at the human dopamine receptor D_4 (DRD4) gene locus. *American Journal of Human Genetics, 74*(5), 931–944.

Xing, Q.-H., Wu, S.-N., Lin, Z.-G., Li, H.-F., Yang, J.-D., Feng, G.-Y., et al. (2003). Association analysis of polymorphisms in the upstream region of the human dopamine D_4 receptor gene in schizophrenia. *Schizophrenia Research, 65*(1), 9–14.

Zhao, A. L., Zhao, J. P., Zhang, Y. H., Xue, Z. M., Chen, J. D., & Chen, X. G. (2005). Dopamine D_4 receptor gene exon III polymorphism and interindividual variation in response to clozapine. *International Journal of Neuroscience, 115*(11), 1539–1547.

VII

Clinical Considerations

18

THE CLINICAL UTILITY OF PSYCHIATRIC PHARMACOGENOMIC TESTING

In order to design more individualized approaches to the practice of medicine, it has become necessary to develop effective methods to clarify the clinical utility of the information derived from the genotyping of specific genes. Studying the pharmacogenomic effects of gene variations in large heterogeneous samples is not a sensible approach to define relatively rare, but still clinically important, associations. This is particularly true when these uncommon gene variants have a profound effect on the clinical course of an individual patient.

The discovery of variants in the thiopurine-S-methyltransferase (TPMT) gene provides an interesting illustration. TPMT codes for the enzyme thiopurine-S-methyltransferase. Only 1 in 300 individuals of European ancestry are poor metabolizers of thiopurine substrates such as the drugs mercaptopurine and azathioprine. Both of these drugs are used to treat leukemia. If poor TPMT metabolizers have leukemia, the potential danger of being homozygous for the low-activity alleles of TPMT is considerable because these patients are at high risk of developing serious, or even fatal, immunosuppression at conventional doses of these drugs. Given this serious medical risk, it would be prudent for physicians to genotype their patients prior to prescribing these medications, to ensure that they are able to metabolize these drugs. However, clinicians were not yet ready to change their practice at the time it was discovered that genotyping could provide definitive protection for individual patients at risk for immunosuppression (Weinshilboum, 2003). Fortunately, this is no longer true.

The Perspective of the Patient

Although some physicians have been hesitant to utilize pharmacogenomic testing, there is little resistance on the part of patients to include pharmacogenomic testing as a component of their care. Patients are quick to understand that the primary benefit of pharmacogenomic genotyping is to identify, and therefore, to avoid or minimize the potential adverse effects that certain medications may cause.

The only persistent disincentive that has delayed the universal use of pharmacogenomic testing has been the cost of genotyping. At the time that the TPMT gene was discovered, genetic testing was perceived to be quite expensive, and many physicians felt justified in their decision to withhold testing because they were committed to minimizing the cost of care for their patients. However, with the development of new molecular genomic technologies, the cost of genotyping has become so inexpensive that it now seems imprudent to take substantial medical risks, such as immunosuppression, to avoid a one-time minimal cost to the patient. We will return to this issue of cost later in the chapter.

The Evolution of Technology

The discovery of the implications of being a poor metabolizer of 2D6 substrate medications provides important insights into the evolution of psychiatric pharmacogenomics. Initially, reports were published of psychiatric patients who were poor metabolizers who developed serious adverse effects while taking a 2D6 substrate medication. However, the results of early research designed to demonstrate the clinical implications of variations in the drug-metabolizing enzyme genes were less dramatic because only a few variant alleles of the CYP2D6 gene had been identified. Over the intervening years, more than 130 variants have been described, including 75 distinctly different alleles.

This explosion in our understanding of the variability that characterizes drug-metabolizing genes has led to an improved ability to characterize the functionality of the wide range of pharmacogenomic genotypes. Yet, since the early CYP2D6 literature was limited to identifying only four or five variants, many subjects were incorrectly identified as extensive metabolizers. In fact, the clinical implications of having an intermediate metabolizer phenotype are still not well established. Unfortunately, even in currently published papers, incomplete or imprecise genotyping can lead to inaccurate conclusions. This was well demonstrated in a reanalysis of pharmacogenomic data drawn from the Sequenced Treatment Alternatives to Relieve Depression (Star*D) trial that addressed an initial report of a negative finding associated with variability in cytochrome P450 genes and response to citalopram. The negative finding was, in part, explained by insufficiently accurate genotyping (Mrazek et al., 2010; Peters et al., 2008).

How Not To Determine Clinical Utility

A good example of the application of older and inappropriate methodologies to assess the benefits of individualized medicine is a report of the Evaluation of Genomic Applications and Practice and Prevention (EGAPP) Working Group (Berg et al., 2007). In 2005, the Centers for Medicare and Medicaid Services (CMS) commissioned this working group to assess the "clinical utility" of cytochrome P450 testing in enhancing the use of selective serotonin uptake inhibitors in patients who had a diagnosis of depression without psychotic symptoms. The working group developed a plan to review what they determined to be the relevant literature related to the potential clinical utility of cytochrome P450 testing in adults treated with selective serotonin reuptake inhibitors. Unfortunately, the approach that the working group chose led to a review of only 37 articles, selected from a potential collection of more than 1,200 articles. The criterion for the selection of these articles was based on guidelines that had been developed for the evaluation of large clinical trials that were designed to demonstrate the efficacy of medications. Not surprisingly, among the selected reports, no large prospective studies had been conducted to explore pharmacogenomic association because such studies are an inefficient way to assess relatively rare associations. The working group chose to reject hundreds of well-analyzed small clinical studies that reveal the relationship between unusual genotypes and unfortunate outcomes. By defining "good-quality data" in a way that eliminated these relevant articles from review, the conclusion of the group was predetermined. Essentially, they concluded that more research was needed to demonstrate the benefit of pharmacogenomic testing. Of course, this conclusion was inevitable because they had not considered the most important evidence that was available to review.

Among the articles that the EGAPP working group chose not to consider was a comprehensive review of empirical data in a 2004 paper in *Molecular Psychiatry* (Kirchheiner et al., 2004). This synthetic analysis of the available literature was based on a review of 342 papers, which included reports from many small clinical studies. Among the papers that the EGAPP group chose to review was a report of 120 patients who were studied while taking paroxetine (Murphy et al., 2003). In this small study, only 15 patients were identified as either intermediate or poor metabolizers. Not surprisingly, this underpowered study did not demonstrate a statistical difference between two quite heterogeneous groups of patients.

In reassessing the appropriate methodologies to assess clinical utility, it is prudent to examine other fields of medicine to compare the rate of adoption of pharmacogenomic testing. For example, in oncology, it has become increasingly clear that the 2D6 enzyme is necessary for the transformation of tamoxifen to endoxifen. Once this fact was appreciated, it quickly led to the discovery that women with breast cancer who were poor metabolizers of 2D6 substrates were being treated ineffectively with tamoxifen. Almost immediately, many oncologists recognized the importance of routine 2D6 genotyping in the treatment of breast cancer patients with tamoxifen and modified their clinical practice parameters.

Similarly, the importance of a report in *Lancet* that described an infant who died because his mother was an ultra-rapid 2D6 metabolizer has led to a rapid change in clinical practice (Koren et al., 2006). The mother was breast-feeding her newborn infant while taking acetaminophen and codeine for pain resulting from her episiotomy incision. Unfortunately, the codeine that she consumed was rapidly transformed to morphine and the infant received a fatal dose of morphine as a consequence of breast-feeding. The original report issued an urgent alert to ensure that mothers who were receiving codeine did not breast-feed their infants without first determining whether they were ultra-rapid metabolizers of CYP2D6 substrates.

There are a number of examples of psychiatric patients who were poor CYP2D6 metabolizers and who died as a consequence of being prescribed CYP2D6 substrate psychotropic medication without sufficiently careful monitoring. Sallee and colleagues reported the death of a young boy who was treated with fluoxetine and developed fatal seizures. Only at the time of his autopsy was it finally established that he was a poor metabolizer and had developed toxic levels of fluoxetine that led to his death (Sallee et al., 2000). A similar report of another patient presumed to have died of a myocardial infarction was determined on evaluation to have had toxic serum levels of doxepin because he was a poor CYP2D6 metabolizer. Unfortunately, the need for pharmacogenomic autopsies has developed as a consequence of the resistance of some physicians to order appropriate pharmacogenomic testing in their living patients (Wong et al., 2006).

COST OF GENOTYPING

As noted previously, the cost of pharmacogenomic genotyping has been an area of some concern. While the initial genotyping of two drug-metabolizing genes was quite expensive and often exceeded $1,000, entire panels of informative genes can now be genotyped for an equivalent cost. Furthermore, most public and private insurance companies have consistently been willing to cover the cost of pharmacogenomic testing for psychiatric patients, when an appropriate indication is provided.

It is inevitable that the implementation of new genotyping technologies will make it possible to very comprehensibly define genotypic variations in many genes at an even more affordable cost. Ultimately, the cost of genotyping will become completely irrelevant, as it is now widely believed that the price for genotyping the entire genome of an individual will be less than $1,000. When this price point is reached, it will not be a matter of whether or not to genotype. The new question will be how to utilize the vast amounts of genotypic information that will be available to improve the care provided to psychiatric patients.

Since 2004, when the U.S. Food and Drug Administration (FDA) approved the Amplichip to genotype the CYP2D6 and CYP2C19 genes, the obvious benefit of pharmacogenomic testing, not only in psychiatry but also in oncology and in the management of pain, has led to the development of more accurate genotyping. In many academic settings, pharmacogenomic testing has become routinely incorporated into clinical psychiatric practice. With the current appreciation of the clinical benefits of identifying problematic variants in the drug-metabolizing genes, the clinical utility of testing for additional gene variations will further refine the ability of psychiatrists to predict the capacity of their patients to metabolize medications. As the clinical utility of pharmacogenomic testing becomes more widely appreciated, the challenge will be to conduct more research designed to further enhance the predictive accuracy of more comprehensive pharmacogenomic panels.

REFERENCES

Berg, A. O., Piper, M., Armstrong, K., Botkin, J., Calonge, N., Haddow J., et al. (2007). Recommendations from the EGAPP Working Group: testing for cytochrome P450 polymorphisms in adults with nonpsychotic depression treated with selective serotonin reuptake inhibitors. *Genetics in Medicine: The Official Journal of the American College of Medical Genetics, 9*(12), 819–825.

Kirchheiner, J., Nickchen, K., Bauer, M., Wong, M.-L., Licinio, J., Roots, I., & Brockmoller, J. (2004). Pharmacogenetics of antidepressants and antipsychotics: the contribution of allelic variations to the phenotype of drug response. *Molecular Psychiatry, 9,* 442–473.

Koren, G., Cairns, J., Chitayat, D., Gaedigk, A., & Leeder, S. J. (2006). Pharmacogenetics of morphine poisoning in a breastfed neonate of a codeine-prescribed mother. *Lancet, 368*(9536), 704.

Mrazek, D. A., Biernacka, J. M., O'Kane, D. J., Black, J.L., Cunningham, J. M., Stevens, S., et al. (2010). CYP2C19 and CYP2D6 variation is associated with citalopram treatment response. *Biological Psychiatry* (Submitted).

Murphy, G. M., Kremer, C., Rodrigues, H. E., & Schatzberg, A. F. (2003). Pharmacogenetics of antidepressant medication intolerance. *The American Journal of Psychiatry 160,* 1830–1835.

Peters, E. J., Slager, S. L., Kraft, J. B., Jenkins, G. D., Reinalda, M. S., McGrath, P. J., et al. (2008). Pharmacokinetic genes do not influence response or tolerance to citalopram in the STAR*D sample. *PLoS ONE*, *3*(4), e1872.

Sallee, F. R., DeVane, C. L., & Ferrell, R. E. (2000). Fluoxetine-related death in a child with cytochrome P-450 2D6 genetic deficiency. *Journal of Child and Adolescent Psychopharmacology*, *10*(1), 27–34.

Weinshilboum, R. (2003). Inheritance and drug response. *The New England Journal of Medicine*. 348:529–537.

Wong, S. H., Gock, S. B., Zhang-Shi, R., Jin, M., Wagner, M. A., Schur, B.C., et al. Pharmacogenomics as an Aspect of Molecular Autopsy for Forensic Pathology/Toxicology. In: Wong, S. H., Linder, M., Valdes, R., Jr., *Pharmacogenomics and Proteomics: enabling the practice of personalized medicine*. AACC Press, Washington, D.C. 2006:311–320.

19

ETHICAL ISSUES TO CONSIDER WHEN USING PHARMACOGENOMIC TESTING IN PSYCHIATRIC PRACTICE

This chapter is written for clinicians who provide their patients psychiatric treatment as opposed to investigators who study their subjects. The distinction is an important one because many reviews of psychiatric pharmacogenomics discuss ethical issues that are important to consider when conducting research, rather than focusing on those ethical issues relevant to the provision of clinical care (Ashcroft & Hedgecoe, 2006; Mordini, 2004; Serretti & Artioli, 2006).

A basic premise of this chapter is that good clinicians often have quite divergent values. Furthermore, these values are contextually shaped by the cultures in which they practice. An interesting example is the contrast of values held by practicing psychiatrists in Great Britain versus those held by psychiatrists in the United States. At the 2008 annual meeting of the Royal College of Psychiatrists in London, a "town meeting" was held to explore "ethical issues" in psychiatric practice. The question formally debated by the group was whether it was ethical to accept direct payments from patients for providing them psychiatric treatment. At the end of the debate, the audience voted on the ethical question. Astonishingly, from an American perspective, the majority of the attending psychiatrists indicated that they considered it to be unethical to accept direct payment from patients. During the discussion that took place after the voting, a British psychiatrist who felt that it was quite acceptable to be paid for his services took some pleasure in pointing out a key irony to the members of the majority. His primary point was that although his colleagues believed that accepting private payments was unethical, they had no problem accepting a government salary, which was provided to them as a consequence of the taxation of their patients.

In contrast to this British perspective, the practice of medicine in the United States has historically and contemporaneously been based on the conviction that it is ethically correct to charge patients for clinical services. Although a wide range of professional opinions exists about how healthcare in the United States should ultimately be financed, I am aware of no American psychiatrist who would denounce colleagues as being unethical simply because they billed their patients for treatment. However, several prominent American clinicians have vehemently argued that it is unethical for a psychiatrist to work for behavioral healthcare companies that "manage" psychiatric benefits, given that these clinicians believe that many of these companies systematically withhold medically necessary care to patients. Given the range of values held by clinicians both within the United States and across the globe, the expectation of a consensus on controversial ethical issues is probably unrealistic.

Fortunately, most of the ethical issues related to the use of pharmacogenomic testing to enhance the treatment of psychiatric patients are considerably less controversial than the thorny ethical issues raised by differential access to medical care based on economic status. Indeed, the ethical issues that psychiatrists must consider when they order pharmacogenomic testing are very similar to those that they have been trained to consider in every other aspect of their clinical practice. For example, psychiatric clinicians have been appropriately sensitized to the imperative that patients' clinical records must be kept confidential.

The primary purpose of pharmacogenomic testing is to minimize adverse medication effects, as opposed to diagnostic testing that may be designed to identify patients who have a psychiatric diagnosis. There will almost certainly be a point in the future when the same genes genotyped to provide guidance in the selection and dosing of psychotropic medications will be linked to estimating the probability that a patient will develop symptoms that, ultimately, may lead to the patient receiving a psychiatric diagnosis. However, this does not occur in practice currently. Rather, any psychiatric patients who would be identified as benefiting from pharmacogenomic testing would have already been given a psychiatric diagnosis prior to receiving the results of this testing. Although pharmacogenomic testing does not contribute to making a psychiatric diagnosis, it does provide clinicians a new methodology that can be used to develop better treatment plans for their patients.

GENERAL ETHICAL CONSIDERATIONS

Four basic considerations help to establish and maintain appropriate ethical practices for the use of laboratory testing designed to enhance the effectiveness of psychiatric treatment. These considerations are relevant whether the data being considered is derived from direct clinical evaluation of the patient, from review of a magnetic resonance image (MRI), from traditional laboratory testing, or from innovative molecular genetic technology (Breckenridge et al., 2004).

1. **Clinical testing must be preceded by appropriate consent.** This has become a guiding principle for all diagnostic and therapeutic procedures. Ethical clinical practice requires that patients broadly understand the basic rationale for proceeding with pharmacogenomic testing and that they have the opportunity to provide explicit consent.

2. **Given the imperative that clinical consent is obtained, it must be clear that clinical testing is a voluntary procedure.** This is true for most laboratory testing, with the relatively rare exceptions of mandatory testing designed to manage conditions that have a negative influence on the public health of the community. Although there are examples of compulsory reporting and monitoring of infections, the creation of these regulations is usually within the context of assuring the health of the public and preventing contagion.

3. **Confidentiality of sensitive medical information must be maintained.** This is true whether the information is derived from a pathological specimen that reveals a malignant carcinoma or from a magnetic resonance scan that demonstrates the atrophy of the hippocampus. Virtually all medical findings must be held in confidence, and the security of the medical record must be protected.

4. **Any medical procedure that is used to establish a clinical finding that will influence treatment and clinical outcomes must be understood within the context of the reliability of the procedure.** The degree of accuracy of clinical pharmacogenomic testing is dependent on a number of critical variables. Certainly two of these variables are the severity of the prognosis associated with the diagnosis of the patient being evaluated and the efficacy of available treatments. In designing the treatment of a potentially lethal condition that may respond well to treatment during the early course of the illness, a laboratory test with very high sensitivity is desirable. The most important objective is to identify those patients who will benefit from treatment, as these patients may not otherwise survive.

RISKS AND BENEFITS

Broadly construed, some risks are associated with virtually all efficacious medical procedures. These risks must be considered within the context of the potential benefits that a procedure may provide to a patient. The evaluation of risks and benefits can result in a considerable range of opinion regarding the determination of the clinical utility of pharmacogenomic testing. If the risk of a procedure is negligible, the potential benefit does not need to meet the same level of professional consensus of benefit that would be the case if the procedure were associated with unambiguous harm.

DISCRIMINATION

For years, there have been legitimate concerns that patients with serious mental illnesses experience discrimination. This discrimination has traditionally been in the realm of reduced employment opportunities, but these patients have also encountered problems related to treatment availability and to the costs of life and health insurance. In the future, using genetic diagnostic testing to identify patients who may be at greater risk of developing mental illness will likely occur. However, this is clearly not the purpose of pharmacogenomic testing, and no credible case of discrimination based on pharmacogenomic testing has yet been documented. Fortunately, this potential risk has been further minimized with the passage of the Genetic Information Nondiscrimination Act (GINA), which went into effect in 2009 (Hudson et al., 2008).

EMOTIONAL DISTRESS

Another risk related to diagnostic testing for any medical condition is the potential emotional distress that may be engendered by the discovery of a pathological finding. This distress is most intense when the illness diagnosed has a poor prognosis. The determination that a patient has pancreatic carcinoma is an intensely distressing experience for both the patient and her family. There is no truly effective treatment for pancreatic carcinoma, and the prognosis is grave. However, it has been determined that it is the right of all patients to receive comprehensive and accurate information about their illness, regardless of prognosis. Today, there is general agreement that to withhold the diagnosis of malignant cancer from a patient is unethical, but only a generation ago it was common practice to deceive patients who had cancer about their diagnosis and prognosis. This same value of advocating for the right of a patient to be aware of her medical prognosis may soon extend to the right of a patient to be aware of those genetic variations that could impact her treatment.

Pharmacogenomic Management of Medications

Psychiatric pharmacogenomic testing is not designed to identify individuals who will develop a serious illness with a poor prognosis. Quite to the contrary, the results of pharmacogenomic testing provide rational and increasingly useful medical information that can be used to protect patients from potential adverse effects of medications.

A current example is the guideline of taking 81 mg of aspirin on a daily basis to minimize the risk of a myocardial infarction. There is now considerable controversy about whether all patients derive a real benefit from this practice (Sanmuganathan et al., 2001). An excellent study showed, for example, that for a large sample of women, taking a daily low dose of aspirin did not decrease the likelihood of having a myocardial infarction (Ridker et al., 2005). However, at a cost of $10 per year, many individuals continue to take daily aspirin in the hope that this simple treatment may provide them some benefit, despite the fact that it may not benefit most people and they are content to accept this cost without pharmacogenomic evidence to better predict whether they will personally benefit. As the cost of treatment increases, the need for more accurate prediction is more compelling.

A Tipping Point

As pharmacogenomic testing becomes more accurate, and as more genes are included in pharmacogenomic panels, the cost–benefit ratio for using this testing to guide psychiatric treatment will increasingly support its application. Moreover, as the benefits of pharmacogenomic testing become more widely appreciated, increasing public pressure for more safeguards in the conduct of medical practice will almost certainly result in pharmacogenomic testing becoming a routine component of psychiatric treatment. This will require the training of practicing psychiatrists as part of their continuing professional development (Marx-Stolting, 2007). Ultimately, if concerns about medical liability continue to increase, pharmacogenomic testing will be viewed as a necessary consideration prior to prescribing psychotropic medications that have potentially serious adverse effects, and the era of selecting medication through a process quite fairly described as using "trial and error" will come to an end (Evans, 2007).

References

Ashcroft, R. E.,& Hedgecoe, A. M. (2006). Genetic databases and pharmacogenetics: introduction. *Studies in History and Philosophy of Biological and Biomedical Sciences, 37,* 499–502.

Breckenridge, A., Lindpaintner, K., Lipton, P., McLeod, H., Rothstein, M., & Wallace, H. (2004). Pharmacogenetics: ethical problems and solutions. *Nature Reviews Genetics, 5*(9), 676–680.

Evans, B. J. (2007). Finding a liability-free space in which personalized medicine can bloom. *Clinical Pharmacology & Therapeutics, 82*(4), 461–465.

Hudson, K. L., Holohan, M. K., & Collins, F. S. (2008). Keeping pace with the times—the Genetic Information Nondiscrimination Act of 2008. *The New England Journal of Medicine, 358*(25), 2661–2663.

Marx-Stolting, L. (2007). Pharmacogenetics and ethical considerations: why care? *The Pharmacogenomics Journal, 7*, 293–296.

Mordini, E. (2004). Ethical considerations on pharmacogenomics. *Pharmacological Research, 49*(4), 375–379.

Ridker, P. M., Cook, N. R., Lee, I. M., Gordon, D., Gaziano, J. M., Manson, J. E., et al. (2005). A randomized trial of low-dose aspirin in the primary prevention of cardiovascular disease in women. *The New England Journal of Medicine, 352*(13), 1293–1304.

Sanmuganathan, P. S., Ghahramani, P., Jackson, P. R., Wallis, E. J., & Ramsay, L. E. (2001). Aspirin for primary prevention of coronary heart disease: safety and absolute benefit related to coronary risk derived from meta-analysis of randomised trials. *Heart, 85*(3), 265–271.

Serretti, A., & Artioli, P. (2006). Ethical problems in pharmacogenetic studies of psychiatric disorders. *The Pharmacogenomics Journal, 6*, 289–295.

20

THE FUTURE DEVELOPMENT OF PSYCHIATRIC PHARMACOGENOMIC TESTING

Psychiatric pharmacogenomic testing has only recently become an important component of the practice of psychiatry, but its future utilization is predicted to ultimately transform the treatment of psychiatric patients. At this time, the primary objective of pharmacogenomic testing is still to minimize the adverse effects of medications in vulnerable patients. However, in the near future, the primary goal of pharmacogenomic testing will be to achieve the now widely discussed objective of selecting the "right drug for the right patient at the right dose." This chapter addresses four anticipated developments in clinical practice that can be expected to occur over the course of the next 10 years. Additionally, it will discuss two substantial barriers that may delay the adoption of psychiatric pharmacogenomic testing and will review a few solutions to manage these problems.

ANTICIPATED DEVELOPMENTS

Development of New Conceptual Models to Better Define Psychiatric Illnesses

In 1980, an important paradigm shift took place in psychiatry with the publication of the third edition of the *Diagnostic and Statistical Manual of Mental Disorders*, (DSM-III). In this edition, all diagnostic categories were based on observable "phenomena." This change required psychiatrists to begin to more systematically catalogue symptoms of psychiatric illness, as it was subsequently necessary to document specific patterns of symptoms in order to establish each specific psychiatric diagnosis. This paradigm shift occurred after many years of practice during which psychiatric diagnoses were inferred from pathological behaviors and were believed to result from "unconscious conflicts" that were the product of opposing impulses, desires, and fears.

Although the more empirically definable taxonomy of psychiatric illness put forward in DSM-III had some clear advantages, its many limitations were almost immediately evident. Most strikingly, a collection of symptoms is better described as a syndrome than as a disease. Many of the diagnoses described in DSM-III included the same common symptoms, such as impulsiveness or fatigue. Additionally, DMS-III provided no explicit way to define symptom threshold levels to be able to accurately validate the presence or absence of key specific disease characteristics.

One of the greatest problems with the 1980 classification system was that patients with heterogeneous sets of symptoms would ultimately receive an identical diagnosis. Although this is true of virtually every DSM-III diagnosis, it is most vivid in those syndromes whose diagnosis calls for the identification of many symptom "criteria." For example, the diagnosis of attention-deficit hyperactivity disorder (ADHD) requires 6 of 9 symptoms of attention or 6 of 9 symptoms of hyperactivity-impulsivity to be present. Based on these criteria, it is conceptually possible for two children to be classified as having ADHD without having a single symptom in common.

Although many problems are related to this heterogeneity, one of the most significant difficulties with the DSM-III, and with subsequent editions (e.g., DSM-IV, published in 1994, and its text revision, DSM-IV-TR, published in 2000), is that their broad syndromic categories do not define discrete phenotypes. Essentially, many DSM phenotypes are so broad that it is highly probable that quite different etiologies are responsible for the development of their symptoms.

To improve the results of psychiatric genetic research it is necessary to define the biological etiology of psychiatric illnesses using more valid criteria. One approach that has considerable promise is the identification of a series of discrete endophenotypes or intermediate phenotypes. An *endophenotype* is a heritable characteristic that can be used to characterize a more homogenous subset of patients. An alternative classification system is one that would identify *intermediate phenotypes*, which are also biologically heritable but represent an earlier prodromal expression of the illness. What will hopefully be achieved in future editions of the DSM is the creation of more homogenous subcategories, based on endophenotypes or intermediate phenotypes, which will replace the broad and heterogeneous diagnoses currently in use.

Definition of the Interaction of Gene Variances to Better Inform Pharmacogenomic Decision Making

There has been a gradual increase in the number of genes that are being genotyped to help clinicians to select psychotropic medications. While the genetic histories of patients have been used to guide decision making for many years, systematic genotyping of the cytochrome P450 drug-metabolizing genes only began at the Mayo Clinic in 2003. In 2004, the U.S. Food and Drug Administration (FDA) approved the Amplichip, which was developed by Roche Diagnostics. The introduction of the Amplichip made it possible to genotype both CYP2D6 and CYP2C19 in any CLIA approved clinical laboratory. Since that time, genotyping of the genes described in this book has become increasingly available at academic medical centers all over the world. However, there is still no consistent agreement about the most effective way to integrate the results of the genotyping of pharmacogenomic panels of informative genes.

It is clear that in the next several years there will be a rapid increase in the numbers of genes that will be routinely genotyped to help guide clinical practice. Some of these new pharmacogenomic "candidates" will be familiar genes, such as the glutamate transporter gene, additional serotonin receptor genes, and other cytochrome P450 drug-metabolizing enzyme genes. However, with the expected exponential increase in the number of genes tested, it will be a challenge for clinicians to interpret the clinical significance of pharmacogenomic testing. It will thus be necessary to develop better methodologies to identify the implications of the interactions of key genes on drug response and thereby facilitate the interpretation of pharmacogenomic testing results.

Identification of the Factors That Regulate Pharmacogenetically Relevant Genes

The history of psychiatric pharmacogenomics is made up of the stories of a series of discoveries that have defined the clinical implications of single variations in genes that influence drug metabolism or drug response. A classic example is the discovery of the Val158Met variation in the COMT gene. Literally thousands of studies have since explored the implications of carrying one or two copies of the more or less active alleles of COMT. Another famous example is the long and short form of the indel promoter polymorphism in the SLC6A4 gene, which also influences the activity level of the gene.

However, it is now more feasible to sequence genes of interest and to conduct functional studies to define the mechanisms by which multiple variations ultimately influence the response of patients to specific medications. For example, in addition to defining the genotype of the indel promoter polymorphism in the

SLC6A4 gene, it may be important to define other variants, such as the variable-number tandem repeat (VNTR) in the second intron and the presence or absence of a single nucleotide polymorphism (SNP) in the promoter region, which is referred to as rs25531 (Mrazek et al., 2009). Based on multiple studies, evidence suggests that by considering these additional variants that influence gene function, a more accurate estimate of the response of an individual patient can be predicted.

Development of Targeted Psychotropic Medications

As the implications of gene variations become increasingly well known, new medications will be developed that target specific patient populations. For example, if a patient has a specific variant of the dopamine 2 (D2) receptor, it will be possible to generate a three-dimensional model of the structure of the receptor and to determine potential functional implications of the variant. Based on this clarification of receptor structure, new agents may be designed to target these receptor variants.

At this time, the process of identifying links between specific drugs and specific receptors is empirical. Individuals with a given genetic variation have been studied, and the likelihood that patients with particular variations will respond to relevant drugs has been documented. However, a more proactive strategy will be to develop new compounds for subsets of patients, based on their defined receptor variability. This strategy has been well demonstrated in oncology, but financial incentives have been insufficient to support the development of targeted psychotropic drugs for small subsets of patients. As drug development technology continues to evolve, this situation will, hopefully, improve.

Barriers to the Adoption of Psychiatric Pharmacogenomic Testing

In the 1990s, there were many barriers to the adoption of psychiatric pharmacogenomic testing. The most obvious barrier was the cost of testing, which was perceived to be quite expensive. There was also far less evidence of the clinical utility of pharmacogenomic testing than there is today. Another historical barrier was that few clinical laboratories were capable of conducting this testing, and the results of testing could not be made quickly available to clinicians.

These barriers have largely been removed by the dramatically decreased cost of genotyping a panel of genes and by the increased availability of clinical and pharmacogenomic testing laboratories across the United States. These developments have resulted in a dramatic decrease in the time required for results to be made available to clinicians. Currently, it is possible for clinicians in any part of North America to receive the results of a panel of pharmacogenomic genotyping in 48 hours. However, two other barriers have persisted.

Persistent Problems in Training the Psychiatric Workforce

Given that pharmacogenomic technology has been largely developed since the late 1990s, psychiatrists who completed their training prior to this point have had little opportunity to master the core knowledge that supports the use of pharmacogenomic genotyping. Unfortunately, there continues to be significant variability in the curriculum provided in psychiatric residencies. A recent survey has documented that, in some psychiatric training programs, the clinical implications of genetics testing have not been effectively addressed (Winner et al., 2010).

Fortunately, this problem of insufficient training has become better recognized at both the national and local levels. It has become increasingly clear that the entire medical workforce needs additional training in the basic principles of molecular genetics. Furthermore, the psychiatric workforce has been identified as a subset of clinicians for whom training in pharmacogenomics will be particularly important. With the creation of targeted continuing medical education training opportunities, an increasingly large number of psychiatrists and primary care physicians will become competent in recognizing the indications for pharmacogenomic testing and in interpreting the implications of these pharmacogenomic results.

Limitation in Providing Computerized Analyses of the Pharmacogenomic Implications of Multiple Gene Variants

Interpreting pharmacogenomic results will become more difficult as more and more genes are genotyped. Hence, another major challenge is the need to develop new technologies that will facilitate the interpretation of multiple genotypic results. The achievement of this goal will require the development of increasingly sophisticated computerized algorithms to quantify the relative implications of multiple variations in multiple genes. While this problem has been recognized for many years, it will become a more critical issue in the near future, as pharmacogenomic gene panels move from sets of four or five genes (Arranz et al., 2000) to large microarrays that can define variability in hundreds of relevant genes. Fortunately, research and development efforts are under way to create computer algorithms that will be able to integrate complex genotypic results and provide comprehensible direction to clinicians.

FINAL THOUGHTS

It is quite amazing that over the span of a single lifetime, the building blocks of our inherited uniqueness have been discovered and new diagnostic technologies are being developed to define the genetic variability associated with both psychopathology and resilience. The birth of individualized molecular psychiatry has been made possible by the emergence of psychiatric pharmacogenomics. Significant advances have been achieved, and the rate of acquisition of new knowledge is now accelerating rapidly. Clearly, there is now good reason to be optimistic that the enormous emotional and fiscal costs associated with mental illness may increasingly be reduced.

REFERENCES

Arranz, M. J., Munro, J., Birkett, J., Bolonna, A., Mancama, D. T., Sodhi, M., et al. (2000). Pharmacogenetic prediction of clozapine response. *Lancet, 355,* 1615–1616.

Mrazek, D. A., Rush, A. J., Biernacka, J. M., O'Kane, D. J., Cunningham, J. M., Wieben, E. D., et al. (2009). SLC6A4 variation and citalopram response. *American Journal of Medical Genetics. Part B, Neuropsychiatric Genetics: The Official Publication of the International Society of Psychiatric Genetics, 150,* 341–351.

Winner, J., Goebert, D., Matsu, C., & Mrazek, D. (2010). Training in psychiatric genomics during residency: a new challenge. *Academic Psychiatry,* 34:2.

GLOSSARY OF GENETIC AND PHARMACOGENOMIC TERMS

Adenine   One of the four nucleotides that are the components of DNA. Adenine is classified as a purine and is also a component of RNA.

Admixture   In humans, the mixing of different ethnically defined groups.

Affinity   The ability of a drug to bind to a receptor.

AIMS   The Abnormal Involuntary Movement Score (AIMS) is a methodology to assess the presence and severity of extrapyramidal movements associated with treatment using antipsychotic medications.

Allele   One of the many forms of a gene that can exist at a single location or locus along the length of a chromosome.

Alternative splicing   RNA splicing is a mechanism by which the exons of the primary gene transcripts are separated and reconnected to produce alternative nucleotide arrangements. This results in the production of isoforms.

Annealing   A process by which two complementary single strands of DNA pair together to form a double helix.

ATG (Adenine, Thymine, Guanine)   A sequence of DNA at the beginning of the coding sequence of a gene that contains the nucleotide triplet sequence of adenine, thymine, and guanine. ATG signals the start of translation within the gene and is referred to as the "start codon" or "initiation codon".

AUC (Area Under the Curve)   The computation of the area under the plasma concentration time curve (AUC), as defined by sequential determinations of plasma concentration, is a method for calculating the relative efficiency of a drug.

Autoreceptor   A receptor located on presynaptic nerve cell terminals that serves as a part of a feedback loop in signal transduction.

Back mutation   A change in the structure of a gene that restores the effect of a previous mutation that may have inactivated the gene. Consequently, a back mutation may restore a gene to normal function.

Base pair (bp)   The combination of an adenine (A) with a thymine (T), or a cytosine (C) with a guanine (G), on the two strands of DNA.

241

Catechol-O-methyl transferase (COMT)   One of several enzymes that degrade catecholamines such as dopamine, epinephrine, and norepinephrine.

cDNA   A single strand of DNA that is complementary to a given sequence of RNA. cDNA is synthesized from RNA by reverse transcription and does not contain any introns.

Centromere   The constricted region of a chromosome that includes the site of the meiotic spindle. This is the heterochromatic constricted portion of a chromosome where the chromatids are joined.

Chromatin   The substance that composes the chromosome and is a combination of the double-stranded DNA and proteins, including histones that compress the volume of the DNA.

Chromosome   A long molecule of DNA that contains a sequence of genes. Chromosomes are visible as morphological entities during cell division.

Chromosome arm   Each human chromosome has a short arm designated as the "p" arm and long arm designated as the "q" arm that is separated by the centromere.

Coding region   The region of a gene that consists of one or more exons.

Coding sequence   The amino acid sequence of the protein product of the gene. Non-coding sequences within some genes include regulatory regions that can include intron sequences.

Codon   A set of three nucleotides that specifies an amino acid.

Copy Number Variation (CNV)   The number of copies of a sequence of nucleotides. Copy number variants may be responsible for phenotypic variability and disease susceptibility.

Crossing-over   The reciprocal exchange of genetic material between homologous chromosomes during prophase 1 of meiosis. Crossing-over is responsible for genetic recombination.

Cytogenetic band   Divided regions of the chromosomal arm that are labeled sequentially (i.e., p1, p2, p3). This counting begins at the centromere and extends toward the telomeres. Sub-bands (e.g., .1, .2, .3) are also numbered from the centromere, extending toward the telomeres.

Cytosine   One of the four nucleotides that are the components of DNA. Cytosine is classified as a pyrimidine and is also a component of RNA.

Deletions   The removal of a sequence of DNA. The size of a deletion can vary from the loss of a single nucleotide to the removal of a sequence of nucleotides that can contain multiple genes.

Dimer   A chemical or biological entity consisting of two subunits called monomers.

Diploid Cells   Cells containing a set of chromosomes composed of two copies of each autosome and two sex chromosomes.

DNA polymerase   The enzyme that synthesizes a strand of DNA as specified by a DNA template. This synthesis may occur during or as a part of a process of repair.

Domain   A discrete component of a chromosome defined as a region. Alternatively, a domain may refer to a discrete continuous part of the amino acid sequence of a protein that is required for specific function.

Dominant allele   An allele that determines the expressed phenotype when it occurs in combination with an allele that does not influence phenotypic expression.

Drug target   A protein encoded by a gene that is critical for the mechanism of action of a particular drug.

Endophenotype   A heritable biomarker that is associated with a clinical phenotype. Endophenotypes may be more strongly associated with genetic variants than are clinical phenotypes.

Epigenesis   The process of altering the phenotype without modifying the genotype. This may involve a change in the properties of the cell that are inherited.

Epistasis   The interaction between genes when the expression of one gene alters the phenotypic expression of a second gene.

Exon   A exon refers to a region of a gene that codes a protein.

Five-prime flanking region (5' FR)   The 5' FR of DNA extends from the 5' end of the sequence to the transcription start site. It is not transcribed into RNA, but may contain elements that regulate gene function.

Five-prime untranslated region (5' UTR)   The 5' UTR is a particular section of DNA that is "upstream" of the start codon of the coding region. The 5' UTR may be a hundred or more nucleotides long.

Founder effect   The cause of a higher than expected allele frequency of a gene in a population. The founder effect is the result of the inheritance of an allele of interest from a common ancestor in a relatively isolated population.

Frameshift mutation   A deletion or insertion that interferes with the normal codon-reading frame. All codons subsequent to such a mutation will be potentially altered.

Gene   A segment of DNA that is involved in producing a polypeptide chain. The gene includes regions preceding and following the coding region, as well as intervening introns between the coding exons. A gene is often referred to as the basic unit of hereditary function.

Gene expression   Occurs as the consequence of transcription and translation and results in the production of a protein.

Gene family   A group of genes that have similar exons. The members of a family of genes are derived because of variations to a common ancestral gene.

Gene cluster   A group of genes that occur in close proximity and are often related.

Gene product   Either a messenger RNA molecule or a protein molecule.

Gene regulation   The control of the production of the functional product of a gene.

Genetic Information Nondiscrimination Act (GINA)   The Genetic Information Nondiscrimination Act of 2008 provided legal protection against discrimination based on genetic variability.

Genetic risk   The probability that a gene will be transmitted or a trait will be expressed in an individual.

Genome   The complete set of genes of an organism.

Genome-Wide Association study (GWA study)   The examination of genetic variation across the human genome. It is designed to identify genetic associations that are linked with observable traits or a disease.

Genomics   The study of gene function or disease expression based on a gene structural variation.

Genotype   The combination of two alleles of a given gene. An individual may be homozygous or heterozygous for a trait.

Guanine   One of the four main nucleotides that are the components of DNA. Guanine is classified as a purine and is also a component of RNA.

Haplotype   A particular combination of genetic variations that occur within a defined region of a gene. This term is often used to describe a combination of polymorphisms that occur within a gene.

Hemizygote   A diploid individual who has only a single copy of a gene.

Hemizygous   The condition of having a single copy of a gene.

Heterozygote   An individual with two different alleles of a given gene.

Heterozygous   The condition of having two different alleles of a single gene.

Histone   A protein component of chromatin that act as a spool around which DNA winds. Histones play a role in gene regulation.

Homozygote   An individual with two identical alleles of a given gene.

Homozygous   The condition of having two identical alleles of a single gene.

Immortalization   The creation of a cell line that is able to be sustained by the process of repeated divisions occurring within a culture.

Imprinting   A change in a gene that occurs during the passage of the gene through the sperm or the egg. The consequence of imprinting is that the paternal and maternal alleles may have different properties in the embryo.

Indel   A contraction of the words insertion or deletion, which refers to two types of genetic mutation that are often considered together, because of their similar effect and the inability to distinguish between them in a comparison of two sequences. In coding regions of the genome, unless the length of an indel is a multiple of three, indels produce a frameshift mutation.

Inducer   A molecule that enhances gene expression.

Inducible   A gene product whose transcription or synthesis is increased by exposure to a molecule that binds to a protein and thereby alters the activity of that protein.

Inhibitor   Molecules that bind to enzymes and decrease their activity.

Insertion   The addition of one or more nucleotides into a DNA sequence.

Intermediate phenotype   Similar to an endophenotype, as it is a heritable trait that may be associated with an illness phenotype.

Intron   A segment of DNA located between two exons. An intron is transcribed and then removed from the transcript by splicing together the sequences of exons that are adjacent to it.

Ki Value   The equilibrium dissociation constant, which is reported in molar units.

Kilobase (Kb)   A kilobase is a sequence of 1,000 base pairs of DNA or RNA.

Linkage   The condition of two or more genes being inherited together because of their location on the same chromosome. The degree of linkage is related to their proximity of the two genes to each other.

Locus   The position of the gene on a specific chromosome.

Logarithm of Odds (LOD) scores   LOD scores provide a method for interpreting linkage tests.

Map distance   Map distance is measured in centimorgans (cM). A centimorgan is determined by the degree of recombination.

Megabase (Mb) 10^6 nucleotides or 1,000,000 nucleotides of DNA.

Meiosis   The result of two successive cell divisions that results in haploid germ cells.

Messenger Ribonucleic Acid (mRNA)   mRNA carries genetic information encoded as a ribonucleotide sequence. The ribonucleotides are "read" by translational machinery in a sequence of nucleotide triplets called codons.

Millimolar (mM)   A concentration of one one-thousandth of a mole per liter which is used to report the concentration of a chemical compound in an aqueous solution.

Molar   Molar concentration or molarity is a measure of the concentration of a solute in a given volume of solution.

Mosaicism   The presence of two populations of cells with different genotypes in a single individual who has developed from a single fertilized egg.

Mutation   A mutation is a structural change in the sequence of DNA within a given gene.

Nanomolar (nM)   A thousand-millionth of a molar concentration.

National Center for Biotechnology Information (NCBI)   NCBI is part of the United States National Library of Medicine (NLM), which is a branch of the National Institutes of Health (NIH). The NCBI houses genome-sequencing data in GenBank and contains an index of biomedical research articles in PubMed. These databases are available online through the Entrez search engine.

Noncoding region   Regions of the gene consisting of the introns and additional components of the gene, but excluding exons.

Nonsense codon   A triplet that results in the termination of protein synthesis.

Nonsynonymous SNP   An SNP in which the nucleotide change reflects a change in amino acid during transcription.

Nucleotides   Chemical compounds of DNA that consist of three portions: a nitrogenous base, a sugar, and one or more phosphate groups. The base can be a derivative of a purine or a pyrimidine. The sugar is either a pentose deoxyribose or a ribose.

Oligonucleotide   A short segment of DNA or RNA, which typically consists of less than 20 nucleotides.

Open reading frame (ORF)   An exon sequence that is translated into a protein.

Phenocopy   Identification of a phenotypic characteristic that is the result of an environmental factor rather than a genetic variation.

Phenotype   A trait or characteristic that is the result of gene expression. Environmental influences can result in modification of the phenotype.

Point Mutation   A form of gene variation that occurs when one nucleotide is replaced with another.

Polymerase chain reaction (PCR)   This reaction is the result of cycles of denaturation, annealing with primers, and extension with DNA polymerase. A PCR will amplify the number of copies of a target DNA sequence by a million-fold.

Polymorphism   An allelic variation that may result in the creation of a different phenotype. By definition, the allelic frequency of a polymorphism must be at least 1%.

Primer   A short sequence of DNA that attaches to a strand of DNA and provides a site for a DNA polymerase to begin the synthesis of a deoxyribonucleotide chain.

Prodrug   A pharmacological substance that is administered in an inactive form, but is metabolized in vivo into an active metabolite.

Promoter   That portion of a gene that is involved in the binding of RNA polymerase to initiate transcription.

Purine   A heterocyclic aromatic organic compound that consists of a pyrimidine ring and an imidazole ring.

Pyrimidine   A heterocyclic aromatic organic compound that contains two nitrogen atoms.

Recessive allele   An allele that is not expressed in the phenotype of a heterozygote.

Recombination   New combinations of genes that are the result of independent assortment and "crossing over."

Reference SNP number (rs number)   Numerical designations created by the National Center for Biotechnology Information (NCBI) to identify unique SNPs and polymorphisms.

Reverse transcription   The process of making a double-stranded DNA molecule from a single-stranded RNA template.

RNA polymerase   An enzyme that produces RNA by constructing RNA chains from DNA templates. This process is called transcription.

Sequencing   The determination of the order of nucleotides in a DNA or RNA molecule.

Silencer   A control region of DNA that like enchancers, may be located thousands of base pairs away from the gene they control. However, when transcription factors bind to a transcription site, expression of the gene they control is repressed.

Silent mutations   Mutations that do not alter the amino acid sequence of a protein product.

Single nucleotide polymorphisms (SNP's)   Single nucleotide substitutions in a sequence of DNA.

Spacer   A segment of DNA that does not have a recognized function. It usually refers to the DNA sequence that occurs between genes.

Splicing   A modification of RNA after transcription. During this process, introns are removed and exons are joined.

Start codon   Sometimes referred to as the *initiator codon*; this is the trinucleotide in a messenger RNA molecule that starts the process of translation. The start codon sets the reading-frame for translation.

Stop codon   Sometimes referred to as the *termination codon*; this is a nucleotide triplet messenger within RNA that signals a termination of the amino acid chain during translation.

Substrate   A molecule upon which an enzyme acts.

Synonymous SNP   A SNP within the amino acid coding region of the gene that does not change the amino acid during transcription. These SNPs usually occur in the third base of the codon.

TATA Box   A DNA sequence found in the promoter region that may be a binding site for transcription factors.

Telomere   The region of DNA at the ends of a chromosome.

Three-prime flanking region (3' FR)   This is the region of DNA that extends beyond the end of the 3' untranslated region (i.e., 3' UTR).

Thymine One of the four nucleotides that are the components of DNA. Thymine is classified as a pyrimidine. Thymine is not a component of RNA.

Transcript The RNA product of a gene that is produced by RNA polymerase.

Transcription The process of copying DNA to produce a single-stranded RNA.

Transcription factors A protein that binds to a site within a gene and influences the process of transcription.

Transfection The acquisition of new genetic markers by incorporation of additional DNA.

Translation The process of protein synthesis that occurs in ribosomes.

Translational initiation codon Messenger RNA is exported from the nucleus into the cytoplasm of the cell, where it acts as a template to synthesize protein in a process called translation. ATG denotes the sequence that is the start codon or initiation codon which begins the coding. The translational codon is usually preceded by an untranslated region in the 5' region.

Translocation The movement of a portion of one chromosome to another chromosome.

Transporter gene A gene that encodes protein can transport a molecule into or out of the cell.

Triplet A codon consisting of three bases.

Untranslated regions Regions of DNA that do not code for proteins. These include the 5'-UTR and the 3'-UTR. These untranslated regions are believed to contain information for the regulation of translation.

Uracil One of the four nucleotides that are the components of RNA. Uracil is classified as a pyrimidine. Uracil is not a component of DNA.

Variable-number tandem repeat (VNTR) The repetition of a short sequence of nucleotides.

Velocardiofacial Syndrome (VCFS) VCFS is caused by a deletion of a small part of chromosome 22. The location of this deletion is 22q11 and the size of the deletion varies.

Wild type That form of phenotype that "occurs in nature." Wild-type alleles usually refer to the most common phenotype in the natural population.

X Linkage The inheritance pattern caused by the expression of genes found on the X chromosome.

Y Linkage The inheritance pattern caused by the expression of genes found on the Y chromosome.

Zygote The cell formed by the fusion of an egg and a sperm. The zygote divides mitotically to create an embryo, which ultimately develops into the individual organism.

Generic and Brand Names of Pharmacogenomically Relevant Drugs

Antidepressant Drugs			
Generic Name	Brand Name	Primary Metabolic Pathway	Secondary Metabolic Pathways
Amitriptyline	Elavil	CYP2C19	CYP2D6, CYP2C9, CYP3A4, CYP1A2
Bupropion	Wellbutrin Zyban	CYP2B6	CYP3A4, CYP2E1, CYP2D6
Buspirone	BuSpar	CYP3A4	
Citalopram	Celexa	CYP2C19[2]	CYP3A4, CYP2D6
Clomipramine	Anafranil	CYP2C19	CYP1A2, CYP3A4, CYP2D6
Desipramine	Norpramin	CYP2D6[1]	
Desvenlafaxine	Pristiq	CYP3A4	
Doxepin	Adapin Sinequan	CYP2D6	CYP2C19
Duloxetine	Cymbalta	CYP1A2[2]	CYP3A4, CYP2D6
Escitalopram	Lexapro	CYP2C19[2]	CYP3A4, CYP2D6
Fluoxetine	Prozac	CYP2D6	CYP2C9
Fluvoxamine	Luvox	CYP1A2	CYP2D6
Imipramine	Tofranil	CYP2C19[2]	CYP2D6[1], CYP3A4, CYP1A2
Mirtazapine	Remeron	CYP3A4	CYP2D6, CYP1A2
Nortriptyline	Aventyl Pamelor	CYP2D6	CYP2C19
Paroxetine	Paxil	CYP2D6	
Sertraline	Zoloft	CYP2B6[2]	CYP2D6, CYP3A4, CYP2C9, CYP2C19
Trazodone	Desyrel	CYP3A4	CYP2D6
Venlafaxine	Effexor	CYP2D6	CYP2C19

[1] CYP2D6 is the primary enzyme for the metabolism of desipramine, which is an active metabolite of imipramine.
[2] These antidepressants are substantially metabolized by other enzymes.

Antipsychotic Drugs

Generic Name	Brand Name	Primary Metabolic Pathway	Secondary Metabolic Pathways
Aripiprazole	Abilify	CYP3A4	CYP2D6
Chlorpromazine	Thorazine	CYP2D6	CYP1A2
Clozapine	Clozaril	CYP1A2	CYP2C19, CYP2D6, CYP2E1, CYP3A4, CYP3A5
Haloperidol	Haldol, Serenace	CYP2D6	CYP3A4, CYP1A2
Olanzapine	Zyprexa	CYP1A2	CYP2D6
Perphenazine	Trilafon	CYP2D6	
Quetiapine	Seroquel	CYP3A4	CYP2D6
Risperidone	Risperdal	CYP2D6	CYP3A4
Thioridazine	Mellaril	CYP2D6	CYP1A2
Ziprasidone	Geodon	CYP3A4	CYP2D6

Analgesic Drugs

Generic Name	Brand Name	Primary Metabolic Pathway
Acetaminophen	Tylenol	CYP1A2
Celecoxib	Celebrex	CYP2C9
Codeine		CYP2D6
Diclofenac	Flector	CYP2C9
Ibuprofen	Advil, Motrin	CYP2C9
Lornoxicam	Lorna	CYP2C9
Naproxen	Naprosyn	CYP2C9
Piroxicam	Feldene	CYP2C9
Suprofen	Profenal	CYP2C9
Tramadol	Ultram, Ryzolt	CYP2D6

Anxiolytic Drugs

Generic Name	Brand Name	Primary Metabolic Pathway
Diazepam	Valium	CYP2C19
Chlordiazepoxide	Librium	CYP3A4
Clonazepam	Klonopin	CYP3A4
Alprazolam	Xanax	CYP3A4

Proton Pump Inhibitor Drugs

Generic Name	Brand Name	Primary Metabolic Pathway
Lansoprazole	Prevacid	CYP2C19
Omeprazole	Prilosec	CYP2C19
Pantoprazole	Protonix	CYP2C19

Drugs Used to Treat ADHD

Generic Name	Brand Name	Primary Metabolic Pathway
Amphetamine	Adderall	CYP2D6
Atomoxetine	Strattera	CYP2D6

Other Drugs

Generic Name	Brand Name	Drug Class	Primary Metabolic Pathway	Secondary Metabolic Pathways
Cyclobenzaprine	Flexeril Amrix	Skeletal muscle relaxant	CYP1A2	CYP3A4, CYP2D6
Dextromethorphan	NyQuil Robitussin-DM	Antitussive	CYP2D6	
Glipizide	Glucotrol	2nd-generation sulfonylurea	CYP2C9	
Glyburide	DiaBeta Glynase Micronase	2nd-generation	CYP2C9	
Irbesartan	Avapro	Angiotensin II receptor antagonist	CYP2C9	
Losartan	Cozaar	Angiotensin II receptor antagonist	CYP2C9	CYP3A4
Nateglinide	Starlix	Hypoglycemic	CYP2C9	CYP2D6, CYP1A2
Ondansetron	Zofran ODT	Antiemetic	CYP2B6	CYP1A2, CYP2D6, CYP3A4
Phenytoin	Dilantin	Anticonvulsant	CYP2C9	CYP2C19
Propranolol	Inderal	β-Adrenergic blocker	CYP1A2	

(Continued)

		Other Drugs		
Generic Name	Brand Name	Drug Class	Primary Metabolic Pathway	Secondary Metabolic Pathways
Riluzole	Rilutek	Glutamate antagonist	CYP1A2	
Ropivacaine	Naropin	Anesthetic, local	CYP1A2	CYP3A4 CYP2C9
Rosiglitazone	Avandia	Antidiabetic	CYP2C8	
Tamoxifen	Nolvadex	Antiestrogen	CYP2D6	
Theophylline	Quibron-T	Bronchodilator	CYP1A2	
Tizanidine	Zanaflex	Skeletal muscle relaxant	CYP1A2	
Warfarin	Coumadin	Anticoagulant	CYP2C9	
Zolmitriptan	Zomig	Antimigraine	CYP1A2	

INDEX

Printed in the USA/Agawam, MA
June 15, 2015

616987.022